OCCUPATIONAL THERAPY:
CONFIGURATION OF A PROFESSION

Occupational Therapy: Configuration of a Profession

Anne Cronin Mosey, Ph.D., O.T.R., F.A.O.T.A.

Professor, Department of Occupational Therapy
School of Education, Health, Nursing, and Arts Professions
New York University
New York, New York

Raven Press ■ New York

Raven Press, 1140 Avenue of the Americas, New York, New York 10036

Made in the United States of America

International Standard Book Number 0–89004–655–7
Library of Congress Catalog Number 81–40372

Great care has been taken to maintain the accuracy of the information contained in the volume. However, Raven Press cannot be held responsible for errors or for any consequences arising from the use of the information contained herein.

Materials appearing in this book prepared by individuals as part of their official duties as U.S. Government employees are not covered by the above-mentioned copyright.

With Appreciation

to the child who bought
    the red loose leaf binder

to the man who recorded
    the marathon

Preface

The purpose of this text is to present a generic or holistic approach to occupational therapy. In this time of specialization, the factors basic to all areas of practice are sometimes ignored or not given due consideration. As a consequence, areas of specialization have, on occasion, evolved without a sense of the common elements that they share with the profession as a whole. Alienation from the profession and identification with a variety of other professions may occur. This frequently leaves the occupational therapist without a feeling of professional identity and the profession without a definition.

A "generic or holistic approach to occupational therapy" refers to the structure and functions of the profession and the way in which these parts stand in relationship to one another. It is hoped that this orientation of the text is reflected in its title. According to the *Random House Dictionary of the English Language*, configuration is "the relative disposition of the parts of elements of a thing." But it would seem that in order to understand the relative disposition of the parts, one must know something of the form and structure of the whole. The same source provides a very accurate word for this, which is *morphology*—"the study of the form and structure of an organism considered as a whole." There was a temptation to entitle the book *Occupational Therapy: Morphology and Configuration of a Profession*. But the temptation was counteracted with the hope that the text would be read beyond the title page.

Structure refers to such components of the profession as the art of practice, philosophical assumptions, ethical code, theoretical foundation, domain of concern, legitimate tools, model, frames of reference, the various aspects of practice and research. Configuration refers to how these elements fit together and influence each other. In addition to structure and configuration, the text also focuses on the content of occupational therapy that is generic to the profession. However, content is considered secondary to structure and configuration. The content of a profession is in a continual state of change. Structure and configuration tend to be somewhat more stable. Thus, the latter, over time, is likely to have greater significance to the reader.

This book is a statement about what is fundamental to occupational therapy. It primarily provides a *groundwork* for understanding evaluation and intervention. Additionally, it illustrates the occupational therapy domain of concern in its totality without regard to areas of specialization. This is not to minimize the importance of clinical specialization, for such differentiation is necessary in any diversified profession. Rather, this volume is an effort to illustrate the essence of occupational therapy as an integrated entity.

I have addressed this text to beginning occupational therapy students with the intention of being a guide through the multiple courses of the curriculum. The content of these courses may often seem like individual pieces of a jigsaw puzzle. Clues as to how these pieces fit together are presented herein. This book is also addressed to registered occupational therapists regardless of their area of specialization or current role. One's perspective often becomes narrow in the endeavor to maintain expertise. There are times in such a situation that a view of the profession in its totality may provide a sense of coherence and direction. Finally, this volume is directed to members of other health professions. The nature and diversity of occupational therapy is sometimes difficult to understand. Perhaps this text will help clarify how the occupational therapist, as a team member, contributes to enhancing the function of each individual client.

Acknowledgments

There are many who contributed to the preparation of this manuscript: Some with full knowledge, some unwittingly, but each in his or her own manner. The list of those who participated is too lengthy to inscribe here. Nevertheless, I am sincerely grateful to them all.

In particular I would like to thank: Wendy Colman, who listened to the drafts in my head; the students in "Theory I", Fall 1978, who joined me in the adventure; Beatriz Abreu, Paula Kramer Goldstein, and Ann Neville, who made copious and pointed comments on the first writing; Deborah Labovitz, who read with critical sensitivity; and Elizabeth Corwin, who dealt patiently with my idiosyncratic approach to the subtleties of spelling and grammar.

To all, again, my thanks.

Contents

Introduction

1 Definition of Occupational Therapy 3
    The Profession 3
    The Client Population 9
    The Settings 12
    The Roles 13

2 Philosophical Origin 16
    Philosophical Assumptions 17
    Ethics 19
    Art 21
    Science 25

3 The Relationship Between Philosophy and Practice: A Loop . 41

The Concept of Model

4 Definition of a Model 49
    An Overview 49
    Structure of a Model 51
    Evolution of Profession Models 52

5 Philosophical Assumptions of
    Occupational Therapy 58

6 Ethical Code of Occupational Therapy 64

7 Theoretical Foundation of
    Occupational Therapy 71

8 Domain of Concern of Occupational Therapy 74
    Age 76
    Occupational Performance 76
    Environment 78

9 The Nature of and Principles for Sequencing the
    Various Aspects of Practice of
    Occupational Therapy 80

10   Legitimate Tools of Occupational Therapy 89
     Nonhuman Environment 89
     Conscious Use of Self 95
     Teaching-Learning Process 97
     Purposeful Activities 99
     Activity Groups 107
     Activity Analysis and Synthesis 113

11   Other Integrative Ideas for
     Occupational Therapy 119
     Common Themes 120
     Paradigm 123

Exploration of Frames of Reference

12   Definition of Frames of Reference 129

13   Structure of Frames of Reference 133
     Theoretical Base 133
     Function-Dysfunction Continuums 136
     Behavior Indicative of Function or Dysfunction 138
     Postulates Regarding Intervention 141

14   Types of Frames of Reference 144
     Analytical Frames of Reference 144
     Developmental Frames of Reference 147
     Acquisitional Frames of Reference 150
     Differences Between the Various Types
     of Frames of Reference 152

15   Additional Comments Regarding
     Frames of Reference 154
     Relationship to Theory 154
     Relationship to the Concept of Model 155

16   Summary 157
     References 159

     Subject Index 167

Section I

Introduction

1/ *Definition of Occupational Therapy*

THE PROFESSION

Occupational therapy, since the formation of its National Association in 1917, has been defined in a variety of ways. These definitions have evolved over time to reflect the changes in orientation and emphasis of the profession. As this is not a historical survey of the profession, these various definitions are not discussed here. Those interested in a historical approach are referred to the literature (2,3,5,17,37,64,65,109,127,130,133,162,166).

For the purpose of this text occupational therapy is defined as the art and science of using selected theories from a variety of disciplines and professions as a guide for collaborating with a client in order to assess that individual's ability to perform life tasks and, if necessary, to assist the individual in acquiring the knowledge, skills, and attitudes necessary to perform required life tasks. Of primary concern to the occupational therapist are individuals whose abilities to cope with tasks of daily living are threatened or impaired by biological, psychological, or sociological stress, trauma, or deficit. Fundamental to the practice of occupational therapy is concern for and use of the nonhuman environment. The nonhuman environment is viewed as an entity to be mastered, an aid to facilitate the performance of life tasks, and a vehicle for assisting in the development of sensory, cognitive, and motor skills and need-fulfilling intrapersonal and interpersonal relationships. Concurrently, the practice of occupational therapy requires skillful execution of personal interactions on the part of the therapist.

The above definition may appear rather vague and sterile. So, to breathe some life into what is indeed an alive and fruitful profession, in this chapter some of the key concepts stated in the definition are elaborated. Many of the concepts are described in more detail in the following chapters. This chapter is essentially only an overview of the profession of occupational therapy.

The first concept of the definition that may need clarification is "art." *Art* is the composition of any artifact or interpersonal experience that diminishes the isolation of the individual; reaffirms the power of the human mind, body, and spirit; and assists the individual in discovering meaning in existence. That which is identified as art assists in fulfilling the universal need for kinship and relatedness to others and the need for a sense of individuality and selfness (28).

The relationship between occupational therapist and client is, by its very nature, one of intimacy. Intimate interactions with others can never be neutral. The therapist's interaction with a client either reaffirms the client's individuality and kinship with others or it denies reaffirmation. The capacity to establish rapport, to empathize, and to guide others to know and make use of their potential as participants in a community of others illustrates the art of occupational therapy.

Although the art of practice is of considerable importance, occupational therapy has also been defined as a science. *Science* is a method of inquiry characterized by agreed upon procedures and rules. It is the process of discovering, verifying, and documenting intra- and interrelationships between the varied components of the human and nonhuman environment. Science is concerned with the analysis and synthesis of sensory data. Occupational therapy is based on the end result or product of scientific inquiry. These end results, in their refined form, are referred to as theories.

Occupational therapists use *selected theories* from other disciplines and professions. The term *selected* is used to indicate that only some theories of a particular discipline or profession serve, in part, as the theoretical foundation of occupational therapy. For example, from the discipline of biology we use theories regarding biomechanics but are little concerned with genetics; from the profession of medicine we use theories regarding the sequelae or consequences of disease, trauma, or deficits but are minimally concerned with the pathological origins. The theoretical foundation of occupational therapy consists of selected theories from the biological sciences, psychology, sociology, the arts, medicine, and theories generated through the practice of occupational therapy.

Occupational therapy is defined as a science because it makes use of scientific procedures and rules to analyze and synthesize data. These data may be gathered through informal clinical observation or through more formalized research projects. Data so gathered are used to assist in the development of theories or to verify, refine, or refute existing theories specific to the practice of occupational therapy.

Occupational therapy is considered to be a *collaborative process* between therapist and client. It is a shared relationship in which both client and therapist have rights and responsibilities. Briefly, the client has the right to be treated as a unique individual and to receive the benefits of the occupational therapist's knowledge and skill. The client has the responsibility of participating in the planning and implementation of a program of evaluation and intervention. In turn, the therapist has the right to receive respect from the client if such respect is earned and to fair remuneration for the application of his or her skills and knowledge. The occupational therapist has the responsibility of acting in an ethical manner and participating in the mutual planning and implementation of a program for evaluation and intervention with the client. Collaboration has the connotation of sharing; of doing with, not doing for or doing to. It is truly a mutual process.

Collaboration, however, is not necessarily limited to the relationship between the client and the occupational therapist. The therapist also has the responsibility to collaborate with other individuals who are concerned with the welfare of the client. These other individuals may be family members, close friends, employers, teachers, or members of the health team. The issue of confidentiality is, of course, important in this aspect of collaboration.

Occupational therapists usually work as a member of a health team. On first contact the therapist explains this working relationship to the client. The essence of this explanation is that the therapist shares all information regarding evaluation and intervention with other team members. This information consists not only of specific facts but also of the client's expressed thoughts and feelings. With the client's understanding of this aspect of confidentiality, the relationship between therapist and client becomes a contract. Thus, for example, when a client says, "I want to tell you about this but do not tell my physician or social worker," the therapist's response comes out of the previously made contract rather than personal feelings or loyalties. The therapist's response is quite simple: "If you do not want to share this particular information with your physician or social worker, then do not share it with me."

Confidentiality and collaboration among the therapist, client, and those significant to the client other than members of the health team are somewhat more problematic. Important variables to consider are age, the client's comprehension, and the understanding of significant others. Two examples may be helpful. It is important for the occupational therapist to establish a collaborative relationship and share information with the parents and teachers of a moderately retarded 5-year-old child. But a 16-year-old girl who is paraplegic may feel far more comfortable discussing her concerns about sexuality with a therapist if she knows that the therapist will not share this information with her parents. Collaboration and confidentiality cannot be reduced to a formula. The therapist's ethical code, good judgment, and wisdom eventually must serve as the guide for being a responsible therapist.

The word *client* as used in the definition of occupational therapy designates the individual involved in a collaborative relationship with an occupational therapist. The client usually is someone living in a community who as a free agent seeks evaluation and intervention through an outpatient clinic, day hospital, or private practitioner. Other terms used to designate an individual involved in interaction with an occupational therapist are "patient" and "resident." The term *patient* usually refers to an individual who is sick: a passive recipient of services. The term *resident* usually refers to an individual who resides in an extended care facility, a halfway house, a single-room occupancy hotel, or an institution that provides care and maintenance for those unable to live independently in a community.

The occupational therapist is and should be involved with those individuals defined by themselves or others as patients or residents. The term client with its connotation of active involvement is, however, preferred by the author.

Occupational therapy is concerned with an individual's "ability to perform life tasks." *Life tasks* refers to all of those activities one must be able to perform in order to meet his or her own needs and to be a contributing member of a community. Thus occupational therapists are involved in helping clients learn to care for their personal needs such as grooming, shopping, and cooking; to maintain satisfactory interpersonal relationships; to participate in the world of work; to engage in satisfying recreational and avocational pursuits. Life tasks, as defined above, are frequently referred to as *occupational performance* in the literature. The latter term is used most frequently in this text.

In the process of evaluation and intervention, the occupational therapist is concerned with "knowledge, skills, and attitudes." *Knowledge* as used here refers to what a person knows or understands about the performance of life tasks. For example, does the client know how to take care of his nutritional needs given his limited budget, does he know the basic behavioral expectations in a work setting, does he know about places in his community where he can meet other individuals who share his avocational interests? *Skills* refers to the actual abilities to carry out tasks. Using the above examples, is the client able to cook a balanced meal, is he able to get to a job on time appropriately dressed, is he physically able to make the journey from home to various places in the community?

To complete the triad, *attitude* refers to an individual's system of values. Values are the degree of worth ascribed to a person, thing, activity, or idea. The words right and wrong, good and bad, should and should not are statements of values. Every individual places some value, negative or positive, on everything in his environment. Thus, again using the above examples, the therapist is concerned about the value the client assigns to eating nutritional meals, arriving at work on time, and meeting compatible people in the community. Values are not always conscious, and some values in an individual's system of values may be incongruent with other values.

"Of primary concern to the occupational therapist are individuals whose abilities to cope with tasks of daily living are threatened or impaired by biological, psychological, or sociological stress, trauma, or deficit." These categories are a broad spectrum of ills to which mankind is subject and include all age groups. Because there is some overlapping among these various categories, some examples may be helpful. Biological stress may be caused by poor posture or insufficient rest. Biological trauma may be a disease process such as cancer or cardiopulmonary insufficiency, or it may be a physical trauma such as severed tendons in the hand. Biological deficit may be inadequate formation of the tissue and bones that support the spinal cord leading to partial or complete paralysis of the legs.

Psychological stress may be caused by worries about money, one's relationship with family members, or lack of a satisfying job. Psychological trauma may include such things as inadequate early parental concern or the death of a parent, spouse, or child. Psychological deficit is exemplified by the individual who is described as mentally retarded or by the child or adult who experiences some type of learning disability.

Sociological stress may be caused by overcrowded housing or community prejudice because of membership in a minority group. Sociological trauma includes family separation due to divorce, war, or migration. Early growth and development in a subculture that does not prepare one to participate in the broader culture is an example of sociological deficit.

Occupational therapists are involved in assessing and providing assistance to individuals who have been affected by the stresses, traumas, and deficits described above. These are, however, only illustrations of the effects of stress, trauma, and deficit with which an occupational therapist might be concerned.

"Threatened or impaired" in the definition of occupational therapy refers to the point at which the occupational therapist becomes involved with a particular client. The term *threatened* refers to preventative measures or to early intervention. Two examples of prevention or early intervention are helping teenage pregnant girls understand the responsibilities of being a parent and assisting youths from high crime rate areas to develop work skills and attitudes typical of the broader society. The term *impaired* refers to evaluation and intervention that take place after some dysfunction becomes evident.

"Fundamental to the practice of occupational therapy is concern for and use of the nonhuman environment." The term *nonhuman environment* refers to all aspects of the environment that are not human: natural objects such as plants, animals, the wind, fields, and mountains, as well as man-made objects such as books, works of art, household furnishings, and computers. The occupational therapist is concerned with helping clients to become adept in manipulating the nonhuman environment. Thus a client may be taught to apply make-up appropriately, tie a necktie with one hand, fill out a job application, or play chess. The occupational therapist uses the nonhuman environment as an aid to facilitate the performance of life tasks. The therapist may provide and teach the client how to use various devices that enhance his independence. For example, a hand splint can be fabricated to allow a crippled client to write with a pen, clothes can be designed that allow a wheelchair-bound child to dress independently, and an amputee can be taught how to use an upper extremity prosthesis.

Finally, the nonhuman environment is used as a vehicle for the development of skills. For example, to assist in the acquisition of sensory-integrative skills the therapist might play with a child on a rocking board that develops his sense of balance; he may engage a client in caring for tropical fish to assist him in understanding the nurturing process. To help a client develop insight, the therapist might use self-expressive activities such as drawing or writing poetry. Involving a group of clients in planning and looking after a small vegetable garden assists them in learning how to take appropriate roles in a group situation.

According to the last part of the definition, "the practice of occupational therapy requires skillful execution of personal interactions on the part of the therapist." The occupational therapist is concerned with promoting the client's growth, development, functioning, and ability to cope with and gain satisfaction from life. This process is facilitated by establishing *rapport*— a comfortable, unconstrained relationship characterized by perception of the client as a unique, knowledgeable person who is worthy of respect and love. The occupational therapist is an intrinsic part of each activity designed to enhance a client's functioning. Through his actions, the occupational therapist stimulates the client's appreciation, expression, and functional use of his own latent inner resources.

THE CLIENT POPULATION

As some of the above illustrations may have indicated, occupational therapists work with individuals in all age groups. Even before a child is born the occupational therapist may influence its development by assisting a physically handicapped mother to devise strategies to ensure safe child care. The occupational therapist provides programs to enhance the neurophysiological maturation of infants who appear to be delayed in this area of development. Parents of physically handicapped children are taught how to hold and position their children to make bathing, feeding, and dressing optimally comfortable for parent and child. A child born without one arm may be fitted as early as a few months of age with a simple static prosthesis.

In such a case, the occupational therapist may suggest a number of activities to promote gross bilateral motor skills.

The occupational therapist frequently cares for toddlers and preschool age children with cerebral palsy. Such children present a variety of problems depending on the severity and nature of their disability. For example, the occupational therapist might be involved in teaching the child how to feed himself, take care of his elimination needs, and dress independently; designing activities to increase muscle strength, range of joint motion, and coordination; assessing the need for a wheelchair with various modifications; or all of the above. Also, the occupational therapist often works with mentally retarded or emotionally disturbed children at this age level. Although theories that serve as the bases for intervention vary, the occupational therapist is primarily concerned with helping the child to develop as many age-appropriate motor, cognitive, and social skills as possible.

In addition to continuing to work with the types of children mentioned above, the occupational therapist whose clients are late preschool and early school age is often involved in intervention relative to children described as learning disabled. Activities and goals relative to occupational therapy for this group include tasks involving interaction with a variety of sensory stimuli such as textures and shapes to enhance tactile discrimination and games which provide vestibular input to improve balance and equilibrium.

Adolescents and young adults coming to occupational therapy frequently are emotionally disturbed or have been injured in some type of accident. The occupational therapist may be initially concerned with helping the emotionally disturbed individual plan and successfully complete a task and to participate adequately in group situations. For example, the therapist might engage the client in a graded sequence of tasks that entail increasingly more complex directions and in a cooking group in which each participant is responsible for preparing a dish to be served at a meal.

The number of possible injuries from accidents is, of course, considerable. One example is severance of the radial nerve. After surgical repair considerable time elapses before the nerve functions normally. Impairment of the radial nerve impedes extension of the wrist and fingers. This in turn may lead to flexion contractures, which may cause permanent loss of range of motion. The occupational therapist treating a client with such an injury would be concerned with providing a dynamic splint and various activities to assist in maintaining good range of motion and adequate strength in the unaffected muscles.

Adult clients of the occupational therapist frequently have cardiovascular disease and pulmonary deficit. One common sequela of both of these conditions is a decrease in the individual's energy level. The occupational therapist is thus concerned with helping the individual learn how to conserve energy through simplifying work. For example, the therapist may teach the client how to make a bed or prepare a meal in a way that requires expending the least amount of physical effort.

The occupational therapist also frequently works with adults who have suffered a cerebral vascular accident. Such individuals experience a number of sequelae that affect sensory integration and neuromotor function. Even after considerable efforts at total rehabilitation, clients may need to use a wheelchair after they return to their home. To assist such a female client, the occupational therapist may visit her home to determine what adaptations can be made to accommodate her needs. For example, furniture in the bedroom may be rearranged so that the wheelchair can be moved close to the bed. Grab bars may be installed in the bathroom so that she can move from the wheelchair to the toilet and bathtub; the cabinet under the kitchen sink may be removed so that the wheelchair-bound individual can wash dishes comfortably.

The occupational therapist also may work with a variety of adults whose needs are not being fulfilled by their current life style. Such individuals may manifest dissatisfaction through debilitating anxiety, child abuse, addiction, depression, and the like. The therapist helps such individuals identify their unmet needs and find ways of satisfying them in the community. For example, the occupational therapist might help a woman find a day-care program for her child, help another person budget his time so he is not overwhelmed by household tasks, investigate various shared recreational activities with an individual who appears to have an inadequate social life, or help another person to become more assertive in interpersonal relations.

The occupational therapist works with members of the aged population in many of the ways that have been mentioned above. But, in addition, the therapist is concerned with helping the individual to maintain a realistic degree of independence and to continue to engage in satisfying interpersonal relationships. For example, in a community center that has a program for the aged, the occupational therapist may supervise a sheltered workshop program; help elderly individuals who can move freely about the community to prepare hot meals to deliver to those primarily confined to their home; coordinate a program whereby the elderly share their knowledge of the community and the world of work with grade school and high school children, or encourage involvement in various political activities. Here, as with all age groups, the occupational therapist seeks to reaffirm the uniqueness of each individual and his potential for being a part of the life of the community.

The above outline of the occupational therapist's involvement with various age groups is by no means an exhaustive list of the various sequelae with which the occupational therapist is concerned. Only some of the more common or frequent types of sequelae are mentioned. Some other areas which are not respective of age include individuals who have experienced severe burns, cancer, or arthritis; individuals who require regular kidney dialysis; and those who have been injured in war or by the effects of enforced immigration.

THE SETTINGS

Occupational therapists work in a variety of settings. The list is rather lengthy, but reading may provide some understanding of the extent of occupational therapy practice. Occupational therapists work in community hospitals; university-affiliated medical centers; federal, state, and city hospitals; outpatient clinics, day treatment centers, and satellite programs sponsored by or affiliated with health facilities (for example, mobile rural health teams, community-sponsored inner city clinics, or crisis intervention groups); facilities concerned with the education, training, and/or care of the mentally retarded (such facilities range from institutions that provide continued care for long-term residents, to special schools, to group living homes in the community, to agencies that provide for or coordinate the special services needed by the mentally retarded individual); sheltered workshops concerned with helping individuals learn skills necessary for work in the competitive labor market or providing permanent employment for individuals unable to compete in the labor market; extended care facilities; public and private schools; private organizations such as the United Cerebral Palsy

Foundation and the National Association for Autistic Children; prisons, special schools, and other correctional facilities.

Occupational therapists are involved in private practice and in group practice. Group practice may be shared with other occupational therapists or with an interdisciplinary health team such as a physical therapist, physician, and psychologist. An occupational therapist in private practice may be the initial contact person of an individual or family who seeks help, or the individual or family may be referred to the occupational therapist by a school system, visiting nurse, employer, physician, special educator, or state vocational rehabilitation agency. In some states, occupational therapists in private or group practice are required, by law, to have a referral by a physician for each client.

Regardless of the facility or setting in which the occupational therapist works, the evaluation and intervention process with the client are similar. The therapist is concerned with identifying and enhancing areas of function and minimizing or eliminating areas of dysfunction.

THE ROLES

The above description of settings in which the occupational therapist works is oriented to direct service—the therapist and client or clients working together. However, direct service is only one role in which the therapist may be involved. Other significant roles are consultation, administration, research, and education.

An occupational therapist may serve as a consultant to many of the facilities or institutions mentioned above. The therapist working in a particular setting may also serve as a consultant to other professional groups within that setting. In the role of a consultant the therapist brings his knowledge of the occupational therapy process to provide information that may assist in solving a particular problem. The therapist as a consultant is not responsible for solving the presented problem—that is the responsibility of the person or group who has sought consultation. An occupational therapist, for example, may be asked by an architect to assist in designing a building to ensure that it is accessible for the physically disabled. A nursing supervisor might consult with an occupational therapist in regard to the appropriateness of various toys he is contemplating buying for the playroom on the pediatric service.

As an administrator, the occupational therapist is concerned with coordinating the work of other occupational therapists and other members of the health team. There are many facets to the administrative process. Some examples may be useful in clarifying this role. One aspect of administration is supervision of staff members. Through supervision, the administrator helps the staff member to solve problems relative to meeting the needs of particular clients and gain additional knowledge and skills for future use. Helping staff members set appropriate goals for the department and to develop new programs is also part of the role of an administrator. In order for a department to function comfortably and efficiently, the staff must feel good about working together even during times of conflict. Administrative leadership is critical to ensuring that the staff work cooperatively and have the necessary resources to assist their clients. The occupational therapist who is an administrator can influence the care of more individuals than the therapist who is primarily involved in direct services to clients.

Occupational therapists are involved in a variety of research projects either as individual investigators or as members of a research team. Research may be a full-time responsibility or only one aspect of a therapist's work. The research in which most occupational therapists are engaged is concerned with validating, refuting, refining, or formulating the various theories that serve as the foundation for the practice of occupational therapy. Through such research occupational therapy continues to be a dynamic profession able to meet the ever-changing needs of society.

The education of occupational therapists is of paramount concern to the profession. As a practitioner, the occupational therapist often supervises the field work experiences of students. Field work provides the student with an opportunity to gain skill under the guidance of a master practitioner. The therapist who is primarily involved in direct service to clients may also, occasionally, teach a course given under the auspices of an academic department of occupational therapy. Such courses may be for students at the basic professional level or for therapists seeking advanced education. Further, the therapist may be active in organizing and presenting a variety of workshops, lecture series, symposia, and the like to share new research findings and ideas with occupational therapists and other members of the health team.

Some occupational therapists devote most of their effort to education. Such individuals are faculty members of a university or community college, who usually have a masters or doctoral degree with a specialization in occupational therapy or some related field. Academic departments of occupational therapy are concerned with the education of occupational therapy assistants, basic professional education for individuals who wish to become registered occupational therapists, advanced education of professionally certified occupational therapists (this may be at the masters or doctoral level), and continued education of practicing occupational therapists. Most academic departments of occupational therapy specialize in the education of individuals at one or two of the above listed levels only. Occupational therapy educators are also often involved in research projects and administration. But primarily they are concerned with education—teaching students the knowledge, skills, and attitudes that will assist them in helping clients to become or remain participants in the community.

Perhaps the somewhat sterile definition of occupational therapy presented originally may now have more meaning for the reader. With this thought and hope in mind, to repeat:

Occupational therapy is the art and science of using selected theories from a variety of disciplines and professions as a guide for collaborating with a client in order to assess that individual's ability to perform life tasks and, if necessary, to assist the individual in acquiring the knowledge, skills, and attitudes necessary to perform required life tasks. Of primary concern to the occupational therapist are individuals whose abilities to cope with the tasks of daily living are threatened or impaired by biological, psychological, or sociological stress, trauma, or deficit. Fundamental to the practice of occupational therapy is concern for and use of the nonhuman environment. The nonhuman environment is viewed as an entity to be mastered, an aid to facilitate the performance of life tasks, and a vehicle for assisting in the development of sensory, cognitive, and motor skills and need-fulfilling intrapersonal and interpersonal relationships. Concurrently, the practice of occupational therapy requires skillful execution of personal interactions on the part of the therapist.

2/ *Philosophical Origin*

Occupational therapy, similar to other professions, is ultimately founded on that area of human concern referred to as philosophy (126,138,139). "Philosophy" comes from the Greek *philosophia*, which means the love of wisdom. Today, it would probably be better to define philosophy as the critical evaluation of the facts of experience. *Critical* is used here in the sense of to examine or study. *Evaluation* refers to defining experiences relative to whether they enhance or impede the growth of the individual and the maintenance of a viable social system. Philosophy is concerned with experience: all that we experience—the individual, society, and the non-human environment.

Philosophers through the ages have sought rational answers to the fundamental questions of mankind. From such basic questions as What is life and what is the meaning of human experience?, they have studied the body, mind, and spirit of man; the structure and organization of the family, the community, and the state; the universe as it relates to and supports life. Questions were asked and answers sought not only to understand the unknown but to determine how best to order human affairs to the benefit of all.

Philosophers continue to ask and seek answers to the same questions addressed since the beginning of human existence. We now know more about the nature of the solar system and the circulation of blood than was known in the time of Plato and Aristotle. But much is still unknown. For example, one of the pivotal issues in the controversy over abortion is What is life? When is an individual alive, and in turn when is human life not viable?

Philosophy is a discipline concerned with a broad spectrum of experience. However, only four areas are germane to the understanding of occupational therapy: philosophical assumptions, ethics, art, and science. Prior to discussion of these areas, however, the statement that "occupational therapy, similar to other professions, is ultimately founded on...philosophy" perhaps needs some explanation. A profession is supported by philosophical assumptions regarding the nature of the individual and the individual's relationship to the human and nonhuman environments. These assumptions serve as the bases for a profession's ethical code and in part the profession's domain of concern and legitimate tools for practice. The beliefs held in common by the members of a profession arise from a set of shared philosophical assumptions. Such beliefs provide a sense of common identity and cohesiveness.

To a great extent a profession's ethical code is derived from the philosophical study of that which is moral and of value in human conduct. Such a code guides the day-to-day conduct of the practitioner. A profession's code of ethics, in addition, forms the basis for a contract with the society to which the profession is responsible.

The art of practice is derived from the philosophical study of aesthetics. A practitioner's relationship with a client is by its very nature intimate and usually sustained over a period of time. Through the art of practice the relationship becomes one of support and concern rather than a mechanical interaction with another person.

Science provides guidelines for the development of a profession's theoretical foundation. Science is related to philosophy in two important ways. Science as we know it today grew out of Western philosophical inquiry. The philosophy of science, as an area of study, critically analyzes the methods, "reality," and application of scientific endeavors.

With this introduction, the remaining portion of the chapter is devoted to a more complete discussion of philosophical assumptions, ethics, the art of practice, and science.

PHILOSOPHICAL ASSUMPTIONS

Philosophical assumptions are basic beliefs about the nature of human life, the individual, society, the universe, and the relationships among these various phenomena. Philosophical assumptions are the point of departure for the formulation of any particular system or school of philosophy. They may be specifically stated by a philosopher or group of philosophers or deduced by the student or critic. For example, Kant and his followers assumed that the individual "can have no *a priori* knowledge of the independent structure of reality." Charles S. Pierce believed that problems could be solved and situations altered by the application of ideas (138).

Philosophical assumptions are beliefs held to be "true" and fundamental; they are considered to be self-evident. Philosophical assumptions are "first premises" from which the reasoning of a philosophical system derives its beginning. They are givens in the logical process (128).

It is important to differentiate philosophical assumptions from scientific theories. Philosophical assumptions are a set of beliefs in the true sense of the word. They are based on something almost like faith, on that which is never called into question. Conversely, scientific theories are always questioned. They are continually subjected to study, through research, in order to test their ability to predict events. Philosophical assumptions are not considered to be testable; scientific theories are developed to be tested. An example may be useful. One of the philosophical assumptions of a democratic society is that all individuals are equal under the law. Although such a belief may not be actualized in the day-to-day operation of our judicial system, it is a belief subscribed to by the vast majority of a democratic society. There are several theories regarding the cause of cancer. Scientists accept few if any of these theories as valid predictors. Research relative to the cause and treatment of cancer continues.

There are various schools of philosophy that may be categorized in a number of different ways. One criterion for classification is the body of assumptions that various philosophers hold in common. As there are different schools, there are different sets of shared philosophical assumptions. The assumptions of a profession are usually derived from a number of different schools of philosophy.

There appear to be three major sources of the philosophical assumptions of a profession. One is the philosophical systems that were paramount during the initial stages of the profession's development. The assumptions of these systems tend to be incorporated into the original statements of the profession's reason for being. Often such assumptions are not clearly stated and are identified only in retrospect. Secondly, a profession's philosophical assumptions are derived from the beliefs of those who are seen as significant contributors to a profession's development. Such individuals may have fostered the profession's growth in a variety of ways. Because of their stature and leadership position, these individuals' personally held philosophical assumptions become part of the profession's collective assumptions. Finally, the philosophical assumptions of a profession are often influenced by social change. During a time of rapid social change a profession tends to review its philosophical assumptions; current assumptions may be reaffirmed or the profession may delete or add assumptions. The change in philosophical assumptions is usually influenced by the prevailing schools of philosophy.

A profession, similar to an individual, needs a set of philosophical assumptions. Such assumptions provide a sense of reality among shifting values and a point of departure for development and action (146). In addition, the philosophical assumptions of a profession have several other functions. One function, mentioned previously, is to influence the ethical code of a profession as well as other aspects of a particular profession's model. Secondly, the philosophical assumptions of a profession provide a sense of identity for members of a profession as well as a sense of stability during times of social or professional change. Finally, philosophical assumptions may facilitate communication with the society to which the profession is responsible. For example, one of the philosophical assumptions of occupational therapy is that the individual has a right to a meaningful existence. This is far different from one of the philosophical assumptions of medicine, which is that the individual has a right to life. In the articulation of philosophical assumptions, each profession defines its reason for being to itself and others.

Each profession therefore has its own unique set of philosophical assumptions basic to practice. The philosophical assumptions particular to occupational therapy are described in some detail in Section II.

ETHICS

Ethics, or the philosophy of human conduct, is the study of that which is moral, good, or of value in life and in action (126). It is the continued attempt to articulate principles of human conduct which take into consideration the rights and responsibilities of each individual. All professions, by their very definition, are guided by some ethical code. Indeed, an articulated code of ethics is one of the characteristics that distinguishes a profession from an occupation. A code of ethics often is developed over a period of time as the occupation becomes and is recognized as a profession by the society it serves. Originally the code is passed on verbally from one generation of a profession to another; eventually it usually is in written form.

Ethics, as a philosophical concern, differs from the social sciences. The social sciences are devoted to describing and making predictions about human behavior, whereas ethics is devoted to evaluating human behavior. However, ethics is not addressed to all human behavior. Ethical consideration is given only to voluntary behavior that affects the basic direction of our living. Most behavior may, nevertheless, under certain circumstances, be subject to ethical evaluation. For example, the act of eating has little moral significance. But if food is scarce, the decision of whether a parent as opposed to a child should be provided with a maintenance level diet has strong ethical implications. The question of who should survive is an ethical issue. Another ethical question, perhaps closer to daily life, is the responsibility of a student to report an observed instance of cheating during an examination. Any act has moral significance if an individual's intent or action affects the rights of other individuals, the institutions of the society, or the physical, mental, or moral development of the individual.

Voluntary actions that are of ethical concern involve the selection of a particular end or goal and the selection of means to attain that end. Thus, for example, it may be considered right and good to conduct research relative to the effectiveness of a particular new type of treatment. However, an ethical question may be raised relative to the research methodology. Is it moral to deny treatment, which is thought to be effective, to one group of patients in order to study the effects of a new type of treatment?

Ethical evaluation of means and ends does not take place in a vacuum. Specific goals and means can be assessed only in the context of a defined situation. Surrounding events must be considered as well as the many possible consequences of the proposed action. Here the question of what is the "greater" good is raised. Is it better, for example, to remove an abused child from his home or to attempt to provide support so that the family unit can be maintained? Ethics is concerned with articulating general principles that can be applied to particular situations. Each situation is unique, and thus the principles which are applicable vary. Ethical principles only provide guidelines to conduct. They are tools for dealing with given events.

A profession's code of ethics is derived from the philosophical evaluation of human conduct. Although fairly stable, these philosophical principles change over time as do professional codes of ethics. The functions of a profession's code of ethics are twofold: they guide the actions of the practitioner and they serve as a contract with the society the profession serves. As a member of a profession, the practitioner pledges to abide by and uphold the ethical code of the profession. In daily interactions with clients and colleagues, a practitioner uses this professional code as a basis for determining the moral implication of all behavior (24,159).

As a contract with society, a profession's code of ethics essentially outlines the value system of the profession. A society legitimizes the existence and accepts the services of a profession only if the stated code of ethics is congruent with the traditions, customs, and values of the society. When a code of ethics is formalized in law, as when a profession is granted licensure by a state, society has the right and responsibility to punish those individuals who do not abide by their professional code of ethics. Whether a profession is or is not licensed by a state, the profession as whole has the right and responsibility to punish those practitioners who do not conform to the profession's code of ethics.

The ethical code of a profession is equal in importance to the philosophical assumptions, the art, and the science of a profession. It serves as the moral guide to practice for the professional. Regardless of the depth and breadth of knowledge and skill a practitioner possesses, he violates the trust given to him by the profession and society if he does not live up to and uphold the profession's code of ethics. The ethical practitioner serves his clients and society with much honor.

Each profession has its own code of ethics. The occupational therapy code of ethics is described in Section II.

ART

Many philosophers have been concerned with defining the generic characteristics of art, of that which is fine or beautiful in human experience. This philosophical area of inquiry is known as aesthetics (138). Typically, one often thinks of art in relationship to such areas of human experience as literature, poetry, dance, music, and painting. But this view is too narrow and does not take into consideration the broad perspective of aesthetic inquiry. Philosophers concerned with aesthetics study artifacts and experiences contrived by individuals, by groups, or by nature relative to a global definition of art. Philosophers consider art to be the composition of any artifact or interpersonal experience which diminishes the isolation of the individual; which reaffirms the power of the human mind, body, and spirit; which helps the individual discover meaning in existence. That which is identified as art helps the individual in fulfilling the universal need for kinship and relatedness to others and the need for a sense of individuality and selfness.

The study of art thus is broad in content. However, for the purpose of this text art is discussed only relative to the art of practice (24,28,105). That is, discussion focuses only on interpersonal relationships that occur in the context of professional relationships. The art of practice is not unique to occupational therapy. It is an aspect of practice important to members of all professions. To clarify, the art of practice is defined as any interaction between practitioner and client that helps the client grow in his relatedness to others, appreciate individuality, find significance in life, accept his limitations, and discover his strengths.

The art of practice is difficult to describe in any detail. It has an elusive quality; the actions and feelings inherent in the process are not easily translated into words. Some attempts seem to be called for, however, since the subject has been raised. First, the art of practice is described in the negative: it is not the skilled application of scientific knowledge, nor is it the desire to help others.

The skilled practitioner is able to make fine discriminating choices of appropriate scientific knowledge and professional skills applicable to the individual problems clients present. Skilled practice is the ability to ask the right questions, to select suitable evaluative tools, and to design intervention strategies to meet each client's needs. However, all of this can occur in an atmosphere in which the client is treated without feeling, treated as something subhuman at best. Discriminate use of knowledge may be combined with the art of practice, but the skilled application of knowledge is not art.

A practitioner may wish to help others who are experiencing difficulty in functioning in one or more areas. This is a noble intention and often one of the major reasons why one elects to become a member of a profession. But such an intention must be translated into disciplined action. It is not sufficient to simply help others. In fact, such help may be more detrimental than instrumental in enhancing function. To elaborate, there is considerable difference in helping a person to eat and helping a person to learn how to eat independently. The latter mode of interaction is far more beneficial to a client. But even that is not art. One can be a systematic and sympathetic practitioner. The art of practice, however, is the additional ability which brings the client to a state of renewed sense of self and a deeper understanding of his place in the community of people in which we live.

Although we experience art, it is, as mentioned previously, difficult to define. Art is a rather mysterious process. Most components of art are unknown to the artist and the participant/observer alike. Nevertheless, some personal characteristics appear to be held in common by those defined by others as masters of the art of practice.

One characteristic is a personal philosophy emphasizing the dignity and rights of each individual regardless of the individual's past or present circumstances or future potential. Such a philosophical orientation is often ascribed to in the abstract but not acted on in daily interactions with clients. It is indeed difficult to respect the dignity and rights of individuals who are severely retarded, who have abused a child, or who reject any involvement in the intervention process.

Another characteristic of the practitioner who brings art to practice is perception of the individual as indivisible, as an entity that cannot be divided into parts or subsystems (135,151). A person as an individual cannot retain human qualities if all aspects of the individual are not taken into consideration. Similar to the characteristics described above, it is easy to speak about a holistic approach in the abstract. The words used in discussing a client sometimes portray a different orientation. One may hear such things as "I have a 'hemi' coming in at 4 o'clock," or "Peters, a schizophrenic, was admitted yesterday." It is true that in study we divide the human organism into subsystems in order to understand more clearly. Through the art of practice one integrates the various subsystems and comes to know a client as an individual. Each client, although sharing much in common with others, is special, unique, and different from all other people. In the art of practice the individual is indivisible.

Understanding of the idea and actualization of the fact that each individual is related to (and embedded in) a configuration of other individuals are also characteristics of the practitioner who brings art to practice. An individual is unique and separate but also a part of a family, culture, and community.

From this relatedness, an individual shares common ideas, values, and experiences. Comprehension of this relatedness is especially difficult when the practitioner and client have dissimilar cultural backgrounds, language, and value systems. Thus it is often difficult to comprehend and appreciate terrorism as a way of life, a woman's totally feministic explanation for lack of job satisfaction, or the refusal of a 16-year-old Vietnamese refugee to learn English. To be able to relate to individuals significant to a client and to accept the client's value system are other aspects of the art of practice.

Another characteristic of the practitioner who brings art to practice is appreciation of the client's relatedness to the nonhuman environment. The client's feelings about the immediate and perhaps future involvement with the nonhuman environment may be influenced by cultural or idiosyncratic experiences or expectations. Clients in clinical settings, which tend to be sterile, are often surrounded by nonhuman objects that have little or no meaning to them or that they find offensive: a plastic drinking glass with a plastic straw, no view of the sky, and thin blankets instead of a favorite quilt. The nonhuman environment can be ominous if one is expected to submit to a number of different evaluation procedures and ingest a variety of unknown medications. Further, an individual's nonhuman environment can be threatening if one is surrounded by splints, a wheelchair, and a vast assortment of adaptive equipment. The therapist who brings art to practice studies and accepts each individual's perception of the nonhuman environment.

Finally, the capacity to empathize with another individual is part of the art of practice. There is a considerable difference between sympathy and empathy. *Sympathy* is an inclination to enter into or share the feelings or interests of another person. In contrast, *empathy* involves entering into the experience of another individual without losing one's own sense of separateness as a unique and different individual (24). Empathy is the ability to feel the pain and joy of another individual, fully realizing it is not one's own pain and joy. The separateness of empathy is important for it allows the practitioner to solve problems, make sound judgments, and interpret with objectivity. The togetherness of empathy is important, for it allows the practitioner to be open to the feelings, ideas, and values of the client.

Even with the above outline of some characteristics of those who appear to be masters of the art of practice, there are still many unknown elements.

Although the majority of practitioners strive to bring art to their practice, it is a difficult if not impossible entity to teach. Each student brings to her initial education a collection of memories regarding personal experiences—interactions with the self, other individuals, and the nonhuman environment. Each student has varying degrees of inner security, knowledge of self, and self-acceptance. Each student has some awareness of how her values and expectations are different from those of others. From this mixture of elements educators and supervisors support and foster the art of practice. The student or practitioner is, of course, not a passive element in this process. The individual who strives to bring art to practice must be able to engage in the often uncomfortable process of learning more about one's self, changing one's self, and gaining knowledge about how one's values and expectations may differ from those of others.

The art of practice is assisting another individual to learn and grow. It is the ability to guide others to know and use their potential, to be participants in a community, to love, to play, to find purpose in life. Once we discover in ourselves or others the potential for bringing art to practice, we can only nurture its growth. There is difficult work in this process, but also joy—for ourselves and our clients.

Without art, the occupational therapy process is only the application of scientific knowledge in a sterile vacuum.

SCIENCE

Science is the fourth component of a profession derived from philosophy. Science as a process and its end product, theory, are not unique to occupational therapy. Thus the discussion in this section focuses on science as a phenomenon fundamental to all professions. In Section II the theories that support the practice of occupational therapy are outlined.

Science is concerned with the critical analysis and synthesis of observable data for the purpose of ordering knowledge and making predictions about the relationship between varied phenomena (13,95,100,114,121). A scientist may be concerned about the nonhuman environment, the biological and psychological nature of the individual, or how individuals exist in and develop social systems. However, science is not defined by the phenomena with which it is concerned. Rather, science is differentiated from other types of inquiry by its unique methods and the way in which knowledge is systematized. The latter refers to the articulation of theoretical systems.

Prior to a discussion of science, the relationship between science and philosophy perhaps needs elaboration (36,54,75,115). Science is related to philosophy in two ways. First, Western philosophy is the genesis of science as we know it in our society today. Our science grew out of philosophical inquiry and became an identifiable method of inquiry only in the seventeenth century. Pre-seventeenth century, philosophy was a fairly direct descendant of Greek philosophy. Philosophers conceived of the universe and its parts as an orderly whole governed by laws discernible through rational thought. Concepts about the rational world were developed from a spiritual or supernatural orientation, essentially inside the mind of man. Thus concepts such as soul, spirit, life, and purpose were projected outward to explain natural phenomena. Explanations were in the familiar terms used in relationship to the self. The appropriateness or acceptability of an explanation depended only on its applicability to a wide range of phenomena and whether it was derived from logical reasoning. There was little or no experimentation.

Conversely, modern science is impersonal, empirically based, and objective. Concepts are developed through observation of nature, not out of the mind of an individual. Events are observed, categorized, and expressed mathematically if possible. The relationship between events is subject to experimentation to ascertain whether these relationships can provide the bases for predicting other similar events. Nature is considered not the creation of an artful mind but rather an entity to be studied and predicted. Admittedly, this is a somewhat abbreviated and narrow view of science. If science is defined simply as study in order to make relatively accurate predictions about events, then we see evidence of science in all known societies and cultures (13). The primitive hunter probably knew a good deal about the movements of the animals he sought for food. The rationale behind Greek physicians' use of various herbs in the fourth century B.C. may be considered somewhat imprecise by today's standards, but the herbs often alleviated disease and suffering.

The major differences between science as it is defined today in the Western world and as it has been practiced in distant places and times are twofold (54,75). One difference is in methodology. Primitive methodology was much less strict and based primarily on trial and error. The use of hypotheses (propositions stating the relationship between phenomena) as a basis for controlled research was not evident, nor was there any extensive statistical analysis of data. The other major difference between the science of today and that before the seventeenth century is that in the latter era that which we call the spiritual or supernatural was considered to be a necessary part of a theoretical system. One would fear for the professional reputation of the scientist today who used volition as one of the pivotal concepts of a theory as to why some animals return to a specific area year after year to give birth to their young.

The second way in which science is related to philosophy is that philosophy has taken on the responsibility of monitoring science. Since the seventeenth century, philosophers have developed an area of study appropriately referred to as the philosophy of science—the study of the methods and structure of scientific knowledge and the relationship of science to the understanding and ordering of human experience. Stated in another way, we often think of scientists as individuals who study their fellow human beings and that which influences human life. Philosophers, on the other hand, study scientists in terms of how they carry out their chosen work and the implications of scientific findings as they affect our lives (107).

Philosophers are concerned with the ethics of scientific inquiry; they have sought to determine the rights of the individual who is a subject in a scientific research project. Scientific studies have often been oriented more toward the enhancement of human knowledge than to the welfare of the individuals involved. Another ethical issue raised by philosophers is whether scientists have the right to continue to study a phenomenon that appears to have a potentially negative impact on a large portion of the human race, for example, germ warfare.

In addition to ethical issues, philosophers of science consider the relationship of science to reality. One of the questions of concern is how and to what extent the methods and structure of science distort reality. Science by definition is designed to discover the common elements of various phenomena. Thus the uniqueness of each individual, object, or event is not reflected in scientific theories. In addition, science deals with only one level of reality. Science, for example, can provide us with some information regarding the age and method of construction of a Bronze Age vessel. It does not deal with the aesthetic quality of the vessel. The question here is perspective. Does science always help us to understand, or can it at times interfere with both our understanding and our appreciation? These and other questions by philosophers of science help the scientist to study, with awareness of ethical issues involved, the possible impact of scientific findings on the social system and the inherent imperfections of the scientific method.

Scientists and philosophers of science are not adversaries as the reader may assume from the above discussion. Rather, they are partners in an adventure of discovery. Scientists and philosophers often look at similar issues such as What is life? What distinguishes humans from other animals? Their methods of inquiry are, however, different. Thus, and probably for the benefit of us all, their answers are different.

The Method of Science

In the above discussion it was mentioned that science is a method of inquiry and involves a specific way of ordering data. Although interrelated, these two aspects of science are separated here for clarity in presentation.

Science as a method of inquiry is characterized by a set of assumptions, traditions, and rules that have developed over 400 years (18,20,28,75, 84,113,144,149,157). Scientific knowledge—unlike knowledge founded on authority, faith, or intuition—is derived from documented evidence. A scientist's credibility thus is based not on reputation or power in the scientific community, belief, feeling, or premonition. The evidence must be there for all to review.

Scientific inquiry differs from common sense. Common sense is knowledge gained through experience unwittingly. In acquiring common sense, the individual learns the relationships among various components of the environment through daily interaction with the environment. The scientist gains knowledge through a preplanned and controlled study of specific elements of the environment (9). Science is based on a predetermined scheme. Deviation from the scheme is not considered sound scientific practice. If the scientist does not gain the information sought as a consequence of planned inquiry, another plan is devised. The new plan is usually based on a reevaluation of the previous plan, continued review of the phenomena being studied, and reconsideration of the theoretical system the scientist is attempting to develop or refine.

Scientific method is public in nature. The process and product of scientific inquiry can be examined by the scientific community and interested lay persons. Scientific knowledge is based on concrete, documented evidence available for public scrutiny. As public phenomena, scientific inquiry and the knowledge thereby generated can be communicated in a fairly direct fashion. The process and findings of science, being self-evident, are able to be conveyed with relatively the same meaning to others irrespective of cultural or language differences (28).

Not only can scientific knowledge be communicated, one of the strong traditions of science is that it should be communicated. The mandate to communicate appears to come from two sources. One source is the assumption that the greater knowledge man has, the better able he is to order his affairs and to participate in the social system. This may or may not be true, but it is certainly an assumption that has influenced Western civilization since the eighteenth century. The second source of the mandate to share scientific findings comes from the scientific community. Scientists are aware that they cannot be maximally productive if they are unable to draw on the resources of past and current scientific activities. Although one's immediate colleagues are important in promoting scientific inquiry, the history of science indicates that contemporary science is strongly influenced by the scientific work of individuals distant in time or place. Although various nations and individuals have at times suppressed publication of scientific findings for political or selfish reasons, the tradition of communication remains strong in the scientific community. Indeed, continuous publication of research findings is considered to be one of the hallmarks of a productive and concerned scientist (28).

Another characteristic of science is that it lays no claim to infallibility. All scientific findings are considered provisional (9). Regardless of how often a particular finding has been verified or the degree to which it has been accepted by the scientific community, the finding remains tentative. All past scientific findings remain open to the continued assessment of contemporary and future scientists. The history of science is, to some extent, a cataloging of discoveries that refute known or accepted theories. In illustration, it was once firmly believed by reputable scientists that man would never split the atom or walk on the moon. There is no such thing as a "fact" in the world of science. All research findings and theories are accepted as only provisional.

The above discussion focuses on science in terms of its uniqueness as a method of inquiry and those characteristics that differentiate it from other systems of inquiry. Science, in summary, then, is the process of discovering, verifying, and communicating the intra- and interrelationships among the varied components of the human and nonhuman environment.

The Ordering of Data—Theory

The ideal consequence of scientific inquiry is the ordering of data: the formulation, refinement, or refutation of theory (9,99,113,117). Such activity is then, in a sense, the end product of scientific inquiry. Formulation of theory is the process of developing a theoretical system either through direct observation or through speculation about possible relationships between events. Refinement of theory is the process of altering a previously formulated theory so as to improve the degree to which the theory corresponds with observed events. Refutation of theory is the process of showing in a logical and concise manner that a particular theory is not congruent with observed phenomena. Not all scientific inquiry leads directly to the formulation, refinement, or refutation of theory. Scientific inquiry often is not immediately fruitful.

Scientific theory is here defined as an abstract description of a circumscribed set of observable events. A theory is concerned with how and under what circumstances those events happen and how they are related. The purpose of theory is to make predictions about the relationship between events. This definition of theory is a bit abstract; some elaboration may serve to clarify.

"An abstract description" is an account of several events or objects without dealing with the unique characteristic of each event or object. Stated somewhat differently, theory is concerned with the common elements of people or things, not with individual details. The variability of individuals and events is, however, taken into consideration in the analyses of data.

"A circumscribed set of...events" refers to the parameters of the phenomena with which a given theory is concerned. How these parameters are defined is essentially up to the scientist who formulates the theory. Thus one scientist may state that a particular theory is concerned with the entirety of small group interaction, whereas another theorist may be concerned only with how leadership develops in small groups. A theory is evaluated by others only in terms of whether and to what degree the theory accurately reflects those events included in the stated parameters. In the example given above, for instance, the second scientist would be required to account for a smaller number of events than the first scientist mentioned.

"Observable events" refers to phenomena people can either directly or indirectly see and share with each other. Theory, however, may be formulated prior to the development of the means to directly observe events that are thought to exist. At this point a theory can be tested only by inference. Thus, for example, Kepler developed a theory regarding the place of the earth in the universe prior to the invention of the telescope. Only after the invention of the telescope were scientists able to directly study Kepler's theory.

"Theory is concerned with how and under what circumstances those events happen and how they are related." A theory describes the relationship among all events contained within its stated parameters. An accounting must be given of each event. The types of relationships vary, but some typical relationships are that A, being one phenomenon, precedes, follows, or occurs at the same time as B, another phenomenon. The term *circumstances* is important here for the relationship between a certain set of events may be altered by different events that impinge on the set. For example, the degree of conformity in a small group seems, to some extent, to be dependent on the number of individuals in the group as well as the degree of the group cohesiveness.

Finally, "the purpose of theory is to make predictions about the relationship between events." *Prediction* refers to the ability to foretell in advance. An example of this basic function is as follows: there is a theory which states that a gross deficiency in vitamin C leads to a disease process known as scurvy. Based on this relatively accepted theory, one is able to predict which individuals are susceptible to scurvy given a knowledge of how much vitamin C is contained in their regular diet or taken by vitamin supplements.

Theory is sometimes erroneously assumed to have several functions other than prediction. One misconception is that theory provides an answer to the question why. The question why is philosophical in nature and not a matter for scientific inquiry. A theory describes the relationship between events and/or objects but does not specify the reason for the relationship. A theory may state that given events A and B and situation X, event C will take place. The *reason* for this relationship is not stated in theory. For example, a theory may state that a person cannot survive for a given period of time without drinking water or eating foods that contain a high percentage of water. This is a statement of the relationship between human survival and water. It does not deal with or purport to deal with the unknown of why there is a relationship between water and human survival. Similarly, we know the distance between the earth and the moon, but we do not know why there is that specific distance.

Another misconception is that one of the functions of theory is to provide the means of controlling phenomena. The application of theory, indeed, allows us to control many aspects of the nonhuman environment and some elements of the human environment. But that is the application of theory and not a function of theory. Thus principles derived from the theory of operant conditioning may be used to help children learn how to read. However, application of theory to practice is not in the domain of science.

Related to the above misconception but an idea less widely held is that theory is designed to help us to determine what is right or good. As mentioned previously, philosophy—not science—is concerned with the study of that which is moral, good, or of value in life and in action. For example, a theory about propaganda describes the phenomenon of propaganda. It does not say whether the use of propaganda is beneficial or detrimental in the conduct of human affairs. A theory is value free. The selection of phenomena for study, the amount of resources provided for research, the protection of subjects during research, and the application of theory are all strongly influenced by individual and cultural values. Most scientists are sensitive to the ways in which various values impinge on their work as scientists. However, the safeguards built into the methods of scientific inquiry isolate theory from the value of a particular social system.

Up to this point theory has been primarily discussed relative to its nature and function. A holistic view of theory can be achieved only by looking at its structure. A theory is comprised of concepts, definitions, and postulates (113).

Concepts are words or phrases that label some similarity between seemingly varied phenomena. Some common concepts are book, street lamp, and desk. "Book," for instance, is a concept because it names or denotes all objects that have certain characteristics such as a cover, pages of paper, a text, and illustrations. "Book" does not stand for or represent any particular book, but rather the collectivity of objects with similar characteristics. A particular book may be labeled in other ways if attention is given to other characteristics. It may, for example, be described as rectangular, red, biodegradable, or a dictionary.

Concepts are abstractions and as such may be stated on different levels. At some level of abstraction concepts provide a system of classification. Color, geometric shape, and weight are three examples of concepts that provide a system of classification. Thus a large number of phenomena can be classified by where they fall on the color spectrum, their congruence with mathematically defined geometric shapes, and their measurable weight.

In the formation of concepts there are two processes. The first process is *conceptualization* or division into categories. The student in learning the content of a particular theory is provided with a previously formulated system of classification. Thus one learns about "defense mechanisms," "connective tissue," and "the socialization process." The process of conceptualization is, however, somewhat different. The process involves a basically naive approach to some phenomena without any preconceived or known system of classification available. This was, for example, the experience of the early anatomists and scientists involved in the study of learning. It is fairly easy to conceptualize in a manner typical to one cultural group or academic discipline; it is far more difficult to conceptualize when dealing with previously unexplored phenomena. Yet such a process is, when successful, one of the major rewards of being a scientist.

The second element in the development of a concept or a conceptual system is *labeling*. This essentially involves providing a name for a characteristic common to a variety of events or an aggregate of objects. The name given to an original concept is ideally one that is not commonly applied to a somewhat similar concept, for that leads to confusion. On the other hand, if possible, the label should have some relationship to the common characteristic being named. Many of the labels for concepts that are a part of modern science have Latin or Greek derivations. This tradition was developed because of the two criteria described above. Scientists seek labels which differentiate between somewhat similar concepts but which also bear

some relationship to the identified characteristic. The tradition is com-
mendable. However, on the negative side, this tradition has contributed to
the proliferation of scientific jargon and the need for students to essentially
learn several different languages.

Concepts can be divided into three different types: simple concepts, constructs, and variables. A *simple concept* labels a characteristic that is fairly
readily observable. Most of the concepts mentioned above are of such a
nature. Although many individuals have difficulty describing a tomato as
a fruit, and the line between animal and vegetable is somewhat indistinct,
most people are able to identify a tomato and differentiate between goldfish
and seaweed. Simple concepts, then, are concepts that are directly observable because of their visual and/or tangible properties.

Constructs are concepts that are not directly observable: they must be
defined in terms of a stimulus-response sequence, by inference. Some examples of constructs are intelligence, need, learning, and anxiety. One, for
instance, cannot observe learning directly; nor can one really know the need
state of another individual. Constructs are used in theory to facilitate description and as such serve a useful purpose.

The third type of concept is a *variable*, a concept that can be measured.
Some examples of familiar variables are body temperature, age, and population density. Ideally, all simple concepts and constructs can be reduced
to the level of a variable. However, this is sometimes difficult, as in the
case of intrapsychic phenomena.

A theory is only as adequate as its conceptual system. Three important
criteria for judging any conceptual system are economy, exclusivity, and
measurability. In regard to economy, only concepts absolutely necessary
for comprehensiveness and predictability are acceptable. It is inappropriate,
for example, to use the terms *nonchalant* and *casual* in describing one
manner of approach to establishing an initial relationship with another person. Only one term is necessary; two terms are confusing.

Exclusivity of concepts refers to the development of concepts that are
sharply differentiated from each other. The concepts body image and self-
concept, for example, in the same theoretical system do not fulfill this
criterion. To illustrate, where do individuals' feelings, knowledge, and
attitudes about their body terminate and their feelings, knowledge, and

attitudes about the self as a totality commence? The two concepts cannot be defined so that they are mutually exclusive.

Finally, the concepts of a theory must ultimately be measurable. Simple concepts and constructs are important, but if they cannot be reduced to metric definition they ultimately serve no useful function. One cannot study that which is not able to be observed. In the theory of operant conditioning, for example, the construct reinforcement is ultimately defined as "any event or act that increases the frequency of a given behavior." A conceptual system that meets the above three criteria is far more likely to provide a basis for prediction than a conceptual system that does not meet these criteria.

The second structural component of a theory is *definition*. A concept can be shared only if it can be defined. Thus in the study of anatomy the concept "hinge joint" is useless without definition. However, with a proper definition (a uni-axial joint that moves to-and-fro in one plane), one can easily recognize, for example, that the last two joints of the fingers are hinge joints. Ideally, the definition of a concept is so clear that anyone can categorize phenomena in a fashion similar to the originator of the concept. Thus adequate definitions of task roles and social emotional roles in a small group provide the observer with criteria for identifying and categorizing specific behavior in a small group.

There are many types of definitions, but the major evaluative factor is whether a definition differentiates a particular concept from all other concepts. A good definition of a concept identifies the higher order abstraction from which the concept originates and delineates that concept from all concepts included in the higher order concept. For example, the definition of turtle begins "a reptile of the order Chelonia" and continues with a description of the unique characteristics of a turtle that differentiate it from any other reptile of the order Chelonia.

Definitions of concepts may be abstract, functional, operational, by example, or descriptive. The concept "transference" is used to illustrate these types of definitions.

An abstract definition describes a concept without reference to specific objects, actual instances, practical consideration, or application. The following is an abstract definition of transference: an unconscious cognitive process characterized by a response to a person in a manner similar to the way in which one responded to a significant individual in one's past life experience.

A functional definition describes a concept relative to the kind of action, activity, or purpose proper to a person, thing, or institution. As defined functionally, transference is an unconscious cognitive process that serves to maintain congruence with past experience and minimizes the fear or uncertainty involved in interacting with an unfamiliar person.

An operational definition describes a concept relative to how it is able to be measured in a quantitative or qualitative manner so that it can be treated mathematically. A variable by its very nature is operationally defined. As defined operationally, transference is an unconscious cognitive process that can be measured by the degree to which an individual responds habitually in a manner congruent with past interpersonal relationships as opposed to stimuli available in current interpersonal relationships.

A definition by example describes a concept by giving an instance of the phenomenon labeled by the concept. As defined by example, transference is an unconscious cognitive process characterized by a response as if all persons in a superior position were one's father.

A descriptive definition of a concept depicts in words or represents in picture or figure what the phenomenon looks like. A descriptive definition of transference is an unconscious cognitive process that makes it difficult for a junior faculty member to discuss personal concerns with the department chairperson.

The types of definitions outlined above were presented in a relatively uncontaminated manner. In actuality, most definitions of simple concepts and constructs are a combination of two or more types of definitions. Some concepts are more easily described by one type of definition than by another type. For example, it may be simpler to define a ladder in a descriptive or functional manner, whereas intelligence may be easier to define in an abstract or operational manner. In given circumstances one definition may be better or more appropriate than another. Definitions are useful only to the extent to which they allow others to understand and identify a particular concept.

Postulates are the third structural component of a theory. A postulate states the relationship between two or more concepts. The type of relationship stated may be hierarchical, temporal, spatial, quantitative, or correlative. A postulate described as hierarchical is, in a way, similar to the initial portion of a definition. Some illustrations of hierarchical postulates are "a lizard is a type of reptile," or "taking a bath is one aspect of personal care." Hierarchical postulates are similar to definitions in that they state that a particular concept can be subsumed under a higher order or more abstract concept. This is a simple relationship but nevertheless important in describing the elements of a particular phenomenon.

A temporal postulate is a relational statement that orders events in time. Such a postulate states the sequence of events. Some examples of temporal postulates are "the regular use of heroin usually leads to addiction," or "after repeated use a pencil needs to be sharpened." Temporal postulates are not an expression of cause and effect. Although causality may be inferred by the reader, it is not intended in a temporal postulate or in any other type of postulate. A temporal postulate orders events in time only.

A spatial postulate is a relationship statement that orders events in space. Descriptive human anatomy, for example, consists in part of a number of spatial postulates. Spatial postulates state the topography of objects in juxtaposition. Some illustrations of spatial postulates are "in order to move an object a wheel must revolve around an axle," or "infant mammals tend to stay close to their mother."

A quantitative postulate is a relational statement that describes the frequency of events or objects. These postulates delineate such relationships as how much, how often, and how many. Some examples of quantitative postulates are "the more frequently a group meets, the more likely the group is to develop a high degree of cohesiveness," or "consumption of protein is lower in underdeveloped countries than in developed countries."

A correlative postulate is a relational statement that describes the "going togetherness" of objects or events. Such postulates state the degree to which objects or events are associated. Examples of correlation statements are "tall people tend to weigh more than short people," or "one-syllable words are easier to spell than multisyllable words."

The types of postulates mentioned above—hierarchical, temporal, spatial, quantitative, and correlative—are the most common types of postulates. There are, of course, other kinds of relational statements. Many postulates are not pure in the sense that they may easily fall into more than one of the categories listed above. Postulates are often mixed and thus described, for example, as quantitative and correlative.

Concepts, their definition, and postulates are the structural components of theory. This is true regardless of the area of scientific inquiry or the content of the theoretical system. Thus the structure of theory in the biological sciences is similar to that of theories found in the social sciences. Likewise, the development of an adequate repertoire of behavior is described by Freud and Skinner in different ways, but the structure of their theoretical systems is similar.

Given the above, there are certain universal criteria for evaluating a theory (9). The primary evaluative criterion is whether the theory allows for accurate prediction of events included in the stated parameters of the theory. The idea of accurate prediction is relative, not absolute. For example, a theory is usually tentatively accepted if it allows for more accurate prediction than any other current theory concerned with the same phenomena. The "new" theory is accepted because it is a better predictor, not a perfect predictor. Theories in the biological and physical sciences tend to allow for more accurate prediction than theories in the social sciences. However, biological theories are, for example, not entirely accurate. Thus in a course in human anatomy the student learns the typical level at which various nerves branch off from the spinal cord. However, when working with a particular client a therapist may find many variations from that which was learned in an anatomy class.

A theory is evaluated through scientific research. In conducting research the scientist is first concerned with the concepts and definitions of the theory. Concepts in and of themselves are not directly tested in research. However, the scientist must initially assess concepts relative to the phenomena of concern. The number of concepts used must be sufficient to deal with the phenomena. The scientist attempts to determine whether there are excessive, overlapping, or redundant concepts. A theory containing such concepts lacks clarity and is extremely difficult to test.

The next step in research design is to define the concepts of concern in an operational manner. Less abstract theories make it easier for the scientist to define concepts in an operational manner. However, this does not mean the concepts of a highly abstract theory cannot be reduced to the level of variables. The measurement of a variable may be simple in that the variable is defined in such a way that, in an experimental situation, it is observed as being present or absent. For example, an individual has or has not eaten breakfast prior to arriving at work. To define the concept more finely, breakfast is described as the consumption of solid food or fluids other than coffee or tea. Other variables may be defined in such a way that there is the possibility of delineating degrees. For example, one may define leadership as "the number of times an individual is addressed directly by another individual in a small group setting," or the range of motion of a particular joint as "the reading taken from an accurately placed goniometer."

Once the scientist has reduced concepts to variables, the related postulates must also be reduced. A postulate, so reduced, is referred to as a hypothesis. The concepts of concern at this point have already been reduced to variables, so that only the relational statement must be converted to operational terms. For example, the postulate "positive reinforcement influences the frequency of specific behavior" might be reduced to "giving praise for words spelled correctly on preliminary spelling tests will lead to more words spelled correctly on the final weekly test."

When concepts and one or more postulates have been operationally defined, the scientist is ready to design an appropriate study to test the formulated hypothesis. When the scientist has gathered all of the information possible from the specially designed study, the data are subjected to statistical analysis. The ultimate purpose of statistical analysis is to determine whether the relationship between variables found in a particular study is a matter of chance or a plausible relationship. By convention, if statistical analysis of the data indicates that 95 times out of 100, one finds the same relationship between the specified variables, the hypothesis is accepted. Hypotheses, it must be noted, are never proven or disproven. Rather, they are rejected or accepted always with the idea in mind that at some future date a rejected hypothesis may be accepted or an accepted hypothesis rejected.

The validity of a theoretical system is assessed through testing a varied number of hypotheses that have been derived or deduced from the collective postulates of the theory. A theory is never tested directly. Rather, it is assessed by observation of observable events which are elements of the phenomena that the theory purports to describe.

The process of formulating theory may begin anywhere along the continuum of formulation in the abstract from personal, unstructured observation to formulation from the data derived through the controlled testing of many hypotheses. The former exemplifies the use of inductive reasoning; the latter, deductive reasoning. Another way of describing this continuum is from armchair or ivory tower to the laboratory or the field. In actuality the development of a theoretical system originates somewhere between the extremes of this continuum. In formulating theory a scientist may be at one or more points on the continuum at any given time. Theory formulation rarely, if ever, involves uninterrupted progress in one direction along the continuum; there is much back and forth movement between the armchair and the laboratory, the field and the ivory tower. Regardless of where one begins, the task of developing theory remains the same: formulating concepts, adequately defining concepts, stating relationships between concepts (postulates), and testing hypotheses.

A quote from Paul Zweig (173; p. 8) catches some of the excitement of scientific inquiry that may be absent from this text:

> A theory is a wonderful thing. Beginning with a handful of mere facts, it moves them about like the tumblers in a lock, until there is a click in the mind and a deep feeling of satisfaction: the lock has opened; the facts have abandoned their lonely oddity and become part of the family of relationships, such as the law of gravity, or $e = mc^2$, or eros, or the death instinct, or other explanatory schemes that, at one time or another, have helped us to make friends with the cosmos.

The reader might feel, at this point, that the text has digressed considerably from the definition of occupational therapy outlined in Chapter 1. The information in this chapter is presented to orient the reader to the philosophical foundation of occupational therapy. On this foundation the holistic nature of the profession is built. Through understanding the philosophical foundation of occupational therapy, one is likely to be better able to understand the profession and its relationship to clients, to colleagues in other areas of specialization or professions, and to the society to which it is responsible.

3 / *The Relationship Between Philosophy and Practice: A Loop*

This chapter is essentially a road map to assist the reader in identifying the relationship between philosophy and practice (28,101,112). Figure 1 illustrates the essence of the journey. But before the territory is explored in detail, a few additional concepts need to be defined.

All professions have a model that serves as the basis for practice. Such a model may be publicly stated or part of the unarticulated tradition of a profession. As used in this text, a model is defined as the typical way in which a profession perceives itself, its relationship to other professions, and its association with the society to which it is responsible. The model of a profession is characterized by a description of the profession's philosophical assumptions, ethical code, theoretical foundation, domain of concern, legitimate tools, and the nature of and principles for sequencing the various aspects of practice (66). A model, then, is a collection of the beliefs, scientific theories, and considered area of expertise of a profession. The concept of a profession's model and a model for occupational therapy are described in much greater detail in Section II.

Although professions have only one model, they have a variety of frames of reference. A frame of reference, derived from a profession's model, provides guidance in day-to-day interaction with clients. A frame of reference is far more limited than a model. It is usually based on only a limited aspect of the profession's theoretical foundation and is addressed to a narrow range of a profession's domain of concern (9). Although the concept of frame of reference is described more fully in Section III, a formal definition may be useful at this point. A frame of reference is here defined as a set

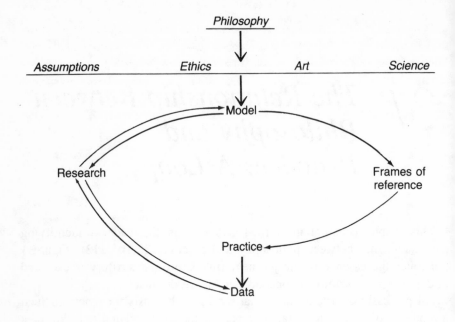

FIG. 1. The occupational therapy loop.

of interrelated, internally consistent concepts, definitions, and postulates that provides a systematic description of or prescription for a practitioner's interaction within a particular aspect of a profession's domain of concern (108).

A frame of reference states the areas of function or dysfunction with which the practitioner is concerned in the evaluation process. It provides an outline of behaviors which indicate whether a client is in a state of function or dysfunction in these specified areas. Finally, a frame of reference delineates the types of interactions, considered to eliminate or minimize dysfunction. The latter is derived from the theoretical base of the frame of reference. A frame of reference is not a formula for action; it is only a guide.

Practice is the application of one or more frames of reference in interaction between client and practitioner (9). A profession's model, in its totality, is only a broad outline of a profession and is not designed for direct application. However, parts of the model are used in the process of practice. Of major concern to the practitioner in daily interaction are the profession's philosophical assumptions, ethical code, and principles for sequencing the various aspects of practice. Practice is the essence of any profession. The roles of consultant, administrator, scholar, or educator are important. But the major function of these roles is to support, enhance, and further refine practice.

Data as used in the context of the occupational therapy loop refers to information generated through practice. The majority of this information is concerned with the degree to which application of a particular frame of reference leads to successful or unsuccessful intervention. Considerable data may be gathered through unsystematized observation. Some examples of unsystematized data are noting that a child is not responding to efforts to enhance sensory integration or that altering one component of a splint markedly facilitates a client's hand function. Unsystematized data if properly considered may provide fertile ground for speculation. Through inductive reasoning such speculation may lead to the formulation of tentative concepts or postulates (168).

The data generated from practice may, on the other hand, be derived from systematic observation. For this to occur, the practitioner follows a predetermined, structured research plan designed to yield specific data. If the research project is well designed, the data generated can then be used to develop, refute, refine, or verify one or more theories that support the practice of occupational therapy.

As the concept and process of research were discussed in the previous chapter, there is no need for further elaboration here. The components of the occupational therapy loop have been at least briefly described. But they have been primarily defined in isolation and not in their relationship one with the other. The term *loop* was deliberately used to identify the interrelation of these components of occupational therapy. "Loop" has the connotation of that which unfolds or encircles in a continuous pattern (152). The arrows in Fig. 1 indicate directionality for this recurrent process.

As mentioned previously, occupational therapy has its origin in philosophy. From philosophy we derive and understand our assumptions, ethics, art, and science. A profession using this philosophical substructure over a period of time develops its own unique model. A profession's model is also influenced by other factors discussed in Section II. However, the philosophical foundation of a profession profoundly affects the origin and evolution of a profession's model. The various frames of reference of a profession are formulated out of the content of the profession's model. If a particular frame of reference deviates too far from the parameters of the profession's model, its use may be questioned by members of the profession and others. Frames of reference provide guidance for practice. Practice, in turn, generates data that may be useful in enhancing the theoretical foundation of the profession.

At this point in the loop, the flow of events ceases to be unidirectional. Unsystematized data, prior to being useful to a profession, must be subjected to rigorous study. This is indicated by the double arrows between data and research. There is, one will note, no direct relationship between research and practice and between research and frames of reference. Research findings influence directly only the theoretical foundation of a profession: a component of a profession's model.

If research findings were directly applied to frames of reference, the theoretical foundation of a profession would, over a period of time, become irrelevant, suited only for historical study. Similarly, if research findings were directly applied to practice, the function of frames of reference as a guide for practice would become obsolete. Taken to the extreme, this process would bring occupational therapy—and any other profession—back to the Middle Ages, when education for a profession was based on an apprenticeship with a master practitioner (66,107). Learning was through imitation of the master and practical experience. There was no articulated theoretical foundation. There was, also, little or no growth in a profession's collective knowledge and skill.

Research findings, then, are first used to modify or support the theoretical foundation of a profession's model. If a particular theory is altered through research finding, this leads to alteration in those frames of reference that use that particular theoretical system. In turn, this leads to alterations in practice. Research, then, is relevant and important to practice, but it influences practice only after findings are incorporated into the model of a profession and appropriate frames of reference.

Finally, the arrows in Fig. 1 indicate that a profession's model may directly influence research. Essentially, these arrows denote a profession's responsibility to continually study its own theoretical foundation. Over the course of its development a profession tends to collect a variety of theories. Some of these theories are in conflict or have been around so long they tend to be viewed as assumptions rather than theory. An alert and progressive profession is always concerned with verifying, refining, and refuting its theoretical foundation. Research related to this process may take place in a clinical or laboratory setting or in the field. Research findings from such studies again are first used to reinforce or alter the theoretical foundation of a profession's model. The findings will in the next phase influence various frames of reference and practice.

In summary, the occupational therapy loop is a schematic representation of the relationship among a profession's philosophical foundation, its model, the various frames of reference of a profession, practice, the data generated by practice, and research. The relationship is continuous, which enriches practitioners and their clients.

Section II

The Concept Of Model

4/ *Definition of a Model*

AN OVERVIEW

The term *model* has many definitions. In general use, model has been defined as "an analogy" and as "a standard or example for imitation" (152; p. 920). In scientific literature, model has been defined as "the orientation and methodology of one discipline used by another discipline as a guide for study." An example of this may be found in Lewin's use of "field theory," borrowed from physics, as a basis for studying intrapersonal and interpersonal dynamics. Also in scientific literature, the term *model* sometimes refers to untested theory.

Sociologists have used the term *model* in two different ways. One use as it relates to medicine refers to the hierarchical social interaction between physician and patient or between physician and other members of the health profession (53,118). As defined by sociologists, the relationship between physician and patient is characterized by the physician being in an all-powerful position. Thus the patient is considered to be "sick," lacking any understanding of medical practice, and thus incapable of making any decisions. A good patient is dependent on the physician, accepts any prescribed medical or surgical intervention, and recovers. In relationship to other members of the health professions, the physician is considered to be all knowing, the repository of all information relative to the restoration and maintenance of health. Other members of the health professions are considered to be lacking in knowledge, inferior, and in need of specific direction by a physician.

However, sociologists have also used the term *model* in a far different manner. It refers to the internal structure and content of a profession (66).

Sociologists' definition of model used in this sense is the same as the definition of model outlined in Chapter 3. To repeat, a profession's model is the typical way in which a profession perceives itself, its relationship to other professions, and its association with the society to which it is responsible. The model of a profession is characterized by a description of the profession's philosophical assumptions, ethical code, theoretical foundation, domain of concern, legitimate tools, and the nature of and principles for sequencing the various aspects of practice (66,94,165).

The above definition is the only definition of model used in this text. The concepts labeled "model" in general use, in scientific literature, and in reference to the hierarchical social interaction between physician, patient, and other members of the health professions are not considered. When the term *medical model* is used in the text it refers to the internal structure and content of medicine as a profession. This is similar to the way in which *occupational therapy model* is used in the text.

Until about 15 years ago the content of the medical model was accepted as similar to the content of the occupational therapy model. Although the content of the medical model was totally inappropriate for occupational therapy in almost every way, acquiescence was not questioned. The reasons for this tacit acceptance are multiple and beyond the scope of this text. However, very briefly, occupational therapy, in its infancy, was somewhat insecure. Similar to other professions in this stage of development, it sought to appear more legitimate through association with a more recognized and powerful profession.

In the mid-1960s, occupational therapy as a profession began to look at itself and at the medical model. Incongruencies were readily apparent (72,81,88). Subsequently, a number of models for occupational therapy were proposed over the course of a few years. Out of this concern for articulating a model unique to occupational therapy the model outlined below was born.

However, before the content of a model for occupational therapy is outlined, the concept of a profession's model may need further elaboration. The structure as opposed to the content of a professional model will be described.

STRUCTURE OF A MODEL

The structure of a model has been previously outlined in the definition of a model. The first two components of a model—philosophical assumptions and ethics—are discussed in general terms in Section I. The other four components need, however, to be briefly outlined.

The *theoretical foundation* of a profession is a statement of selected theories from various fields of inquiry which serve as the scientific base for practice. These theories may be drawn from various disciplines, other professions, and from research findings generated by the profession itself (147). In the past one of the hallmarks of a profession, as identified by sociologists, was the uniqueness of the profession's theoretical foundation (42,46,53, 69,82,107,141,160). In other words, an occupation could not be considered a profession unless it had a theoretical foundation different in its totality from the theoretical foundation of any other profession. Whether this was ever true in the past is highly questionable. And there is considerable evidence to indicate that it is not true now. For example, lawyers use various psychological theories, and medicine would not exist as we know it today without the theories generated by physiologists. The theoretical foundation of a profession must, indeed, be known and structured. In its totality it is unique; its various elements are often shared with other professions.

A profession's *domain of concern* consists of those areas of human experience in which practitioners of the profession offer assistance to others. The domain of concern of a profession is essentially a statement of what the profession believes is its area of expertise. Such expertise is usually recognized by the society to which the profession is responsible. Indeed, the domain of concern is often that component of a profession which is most known or recognized by lay persons. For example, the domains of concern of dentistry and law are rarely confused. There are specialized areas in the majority of professions which are elaborated or further defined in the various frames of reference of a profession. The domain of concern outlined in a model simply describes in general terms a profession's areas of expertise. The parameters of a profession's domain of concern may overlap in some areas with the parameters of the domain of concern of another profession. For example, both the nurse and the recreational therapist are interested in enhancing the independence of a physically handicapped child. However, their specific goals and means may vary. One advantage of the overlapping of domains of concern of related professions is that it facilitates communication between the involved practitioners in regard to particular areas of human experience.

The nature of and principles for sequencing the various aspects of practice refers to the way in which a profession defines and identifies problems and proceeds to solve them. The principles, outlined in the profession's model, provide guidelines as to how the practitioner approaches, assesses, and intervenes. These guidelines are general and do not deal with specific components of the profession's domain of concern, evaluative tools, or procedures used in assisting particular categories of clients. This more detailed information is included in a profession's frames of reference. Principles for sequencing the various aspects of practice simply provide guidelines for an orderly, step-by-step process that ideally leads to enhancing a client's ability to interact in the community.

The final component of the model for a profession is *legitimate tools*, the permissible means by which the practitioners of a given profession fulfill their responsibility to society. Legitimate or permissible is used here in the sense that the profession, over an extended period of time, has demonstrated knowledge and expertise in the use of particular tools. The concept of tools is used in a general sense to include nonhuman objects such as drugs or splints, techniques of interaction such as surgery or providing support, and methods of evaluation such as X-ray or the Stanford-Binet test for intelligence. Legitimate tools may be shared by more than one profession. For example, the professions of social work and clinical psychology both identify verbal psychotherapy as one of their legitimate tools. A practitioner who uses tools not delineated in the model of his or her profession is usually considered highly deviant by members of the profession and society. Such an individual may ultimately be subject to various negative sanctions.

The structure of a model is similar for all professions; the content of each profession's model differentiates one profession from another. Professional models are not, however, stagnant but evolve with time.

EVOLUTION OF PROFESSIONAL MODELS

It seems appropriate to begin this portion of the chapter with a description of the origin of the content of a profession's model. Unfortunately, a search of the literature provided no information in this area. Thus the following brief comments are conjecture only. It appears that the content of a profession's model originates from some vague idea of philosophical assumptions, domain of concern, and legitimate tools. These ideas often are not well articulated but rather are shared at the level of "belief" or joint understanding by the founders of the profession. As the number of practitioners of a profession increases, statements must be refined for two reasons. As the number of students increases, a distance in time and place is created between current students and the founders of the profession. Students can no longer learn directly from the originators. Eventually, in the interest of both adequate socialization into the profession and quality education, a profession begins to articulate the content of its model precisely. The other reason for a more concise statement of the content of a profession's model is the questions raised by society. A profession cannot exist without some degree of recognition and acceptance by society (13,136,147). Essentially, society asks how a particular profession can enhance the quality of life of community members. Or, stated a bit less elegantly, society asks why it should pay for the services rendered by a particular emerging profession (168). In negotiating with society for support, a profession is required to articulate its rationale, goals, and means in a manner understandable to members of the society.

Thus over a period of time a profession begins to state its philosophical assumptions, domain of concern, and legitimate tools more clearly. In addition, an emerging profession slowly addresses itself to the other components of a professional mode. The latter components are eventually described both to facilitate the educational process and to maintain the broad support of society.

One additional factor is important in the process of formulating the content of a profession's model: the need of the members of a profession to develop and define their own identity. This need is similar to that of an individual. All of us, in order to experience ourselves as separate and unique persons, need a sense of who we are, what we are, and why we are the kinds of persons we are. Without a sense of identity, the individual experiences discomfort and difficulty in relating to others. The same is true for a profession.

Although the process of how a profession develops the content of its model is not particularly clear, we do know that at some point a profession and the contents of its model become almost inseparable. Once accepted by an emerging profession and the society to which it is responsible, a model defines and delineates the nature of the profession. The model of a profession after this point in its evolution is rarely questioned by society as a whole. For example, we expect a dentist to do something positive about a toothache, we expect a journalist to provide an unbiased report of daily events. Neither of these examples may be accurate relative to a particular practitioner; nevertheless, these are our expectations for a profession as a whole. These expectations simply grow out of our understanding of the model of the exemplified professions.

Similarly, at this point in its evolution, a model, in its totality, is rarely questioned by members of the profession. There is a general acceptance of the content of the model. This is not to say that members of a profession do not periodically reassess specific aspects of their model; yet the gestalt of the model is not questioned. Even the revolutionary social forces of the late 1960s and early 1970s, which engulfed most professions, left behind few major changes in the models of the professions.

Once defined, however, the model of a profession is not static. Its content is continually in flux, but this change is not necessarily undirected. Professions have a "filter" for selecting theoretical data significant to practice. This filter provides guidelines for the profession in selecting, categorizing, and using data generated by scientific inquiry (54,87,94,121). The data generated through research in the various disciplines and professions are considerable. Only certain data, however, are useful to a particular profession. For example, an astronomer is interested in data relative to the phenomena of black holes. A physical therapist, although perhaps interested in such information as an individual, would not consider such data pertinent to the theoretical foundation of physical therapy. Moreover, data identified as important by two or more professions may be interpreted, processed, and used differently by those professions. For example, a newspaper publisher and a sociologist use data gathered from demographic studies in somewhat dissimilar manners.

The criteria or guidelines for selecting data pertinent to a profession are influenced by the current theoretical foundation, domain of concern, and legitimate tools of the profession. Essentially, in the survey of available data a profession asks, "Will these data enhance the ability of practitioners to fulfill their contract with society?" Each profession selects information important for substantiating, refining, or altering the content of its model. Some information generated by scientific inquiry is considered germane, other information is considered irrelevant.

Change in a profession's model may be so gradual that it is hardly noticed by the members of the profession or by others. At other times the change may be so rapid that it is considered revolutionary. One of the classic examples of the latter situation is the introduction of antibiotics as one of the legitimate tools of medicine. This not only altered the course of many disease processes but contributed greatly to the well-being of society.

The contents of a profession's model that appear to change in the most obvious manner are a model's domain of concern and legitimate tools. An example in regard to legitimate tools is provided in the above paragraph. An example of a somewhat dramatic change in domain of concern can be seen in education. Only in fairly recent years have educators identified the individual with "learning disabilities" as one aspect of their domain of concern.

Changes in a profession's domain of concern and legitimate tools are fairly evident to the lay person. But change in one component often leads to changes in other components. For example, alteration in a model's domain of concern or legitimate tools can rarely be accommodated without some alteration in a profession's theoretical foundation. The model of a profession is similar in many ways to a social system. Change in one area reverberates throughout the system (118). In illustration, the role of women in Western society appears to be in a process of redefinition. This redefinition has affected many other components of various social systems. The same is true relative to the model of a profession.

The evolution of a profession's model appears to be influenced by three factors. Scientific information from outside the profession may bring about change. An example of this can be seen in physical therapy's inclusion of biofeedback as one of its legitimate tools. The second factor is scientific information generated internally. Skinner's theory of operant conditioning, for example, has greatly influenced the discipline and profession of psychology. The third factor is a vacuum in services identified by the society to which a profession is responsible (141). Although societies may support the development of a new profession to fulfill newly identified needs, more typically societies first seek the assistance of their existing professions. For example, when the extent and severity of the problems of learning disabled children and adults became apparent to our society help was sought from educators and various health professionals.

Conversely, the evolution of a profession's model is restrained by several factors. First is the inherent traditionalism of a profession. Over a period of years, professions often tend to become somewhat inflexible and suspicious of that which is new or different. A classic example of this is education's hesitancy in using videotaped lectures as the primary source of instruction in higher education.

The general knowledge and expertise of a profession is another restraining factor. A profession puts itself at great risk if it attempts to interact in an area of human experience without sufficient skill or understanding. Obviously, such interaction may be harmful to clients. In addition, it is often detrimental to the reputation of the profession. Thus a responsible profession does not move into a new area without first determining whether a sufficient portion of its members have adequate comprehension of the task to be accomplished. A profession takes many risks in promising more than it can deliver.

The third restraint to the evolution of a profession's model is the content of the model of other professions. Professions tend to be possessive in regard to the content of their model and are not prone to sharing with other professions. Indeed, although there are many reasons for licensure laws, one of the reasons is to protect a profession's "territory" from other professions. Two components of a profession's model that seem to be the most jealously guarded are domain of concern and legitimate tools. An example of this relative to domain of concern can be seen in the ongoing discussion between nurses and physician assistants as to each of their appropriate roles and functions in a clinical setting.

The final major restraint on the evolution of a profession's model is the society or societies to which the profession is responsible. Ultimately, society determines the validity of a profession. Without the moral and financial support of society a profession cannot exist. In addition, society to a great extent determines the differing responsibilities of each profession. In for-

mulating and altering the content of its model a profession essentially ne-
gotiates with society. Such negotiation tends to be an ongoing dialogue
(71,141). Accountability is probably the key factor in this dialogue. Society
asks for services of one kind or another and demands evidence that those
services have been successfully rendered. A profession, in turn, defines its
various areas of expertise and attempts to demonstrate a high degree of
problem resolution.

In summary, the concept *model*, as used in this text, is the typical way
in which a profession perceives itself, its relationship to other professions,
and its association with the society to which it is responsible. The structure
or components of a model are similar for all professions. Although some
of the content of a profession's model may be shared with other professions,
in its totality each profession's model is unique. Once a model is accepted
by a profession, it tends to remain relatively stable over time. Nevertheless,
a profession's model has a propensity to evolve and change. Several factors,
described above, both contribute to and restrain the evolution of a profession's model. The model of a profession reflects a combination of the
profession's areas and levels of expertise as defined by the profession and
the acceptance of that definition by other professions and society.

The following chapters in this section describe a model for occupational
therapy. The content of this model in its totality is not accepted by all
members of the profession. Because occupational therapy is an emerging
profession, the content of its model remains in flux, somewhat tentative in
nature. Thus these subsequent chapters should be read in an exploratory and
critical manner.

As the components of the occupational therapy model are described, the
content of the medical model is used as a means of clarification (30,53,
129,130,136,137,147,155,170). However, the content of the medical model
is not described in any great detail. The medical model was selected for
illustration because it was felt that the reader is likely to be more familiar
with its content than with the content of the models of other professions.

5 / *Philosophical Assumptions of Occupational Therapy*

Philosophical assumptions are basic beliefs about the nature of human life, the individual, society, the universe, and the relationships among these various elements. The philosophical assumptions of a profession state how the members of the profession view the individual as an individual and his or her interrelatedness with the human and nonhuman environments. Further, the philosophical assumptions of a profession provide a substructure for the other components of a profession's model (66).

In 1979 the American Occupational Therapy Delegate Assembly adopted the following statement of "The Philosophical Base of Occupational Therapy":

> Man is an active being whose development is influenced by the use of purposeful activity. Using their capacity for intrinsic motivation, human beings are able to influence their physical and mental health and their social and physical environment through purposeful activity. Human life includes a process of continuous adaptation. Adaptation is a change in function that promotes survival and self-actualization. Biological, psychological, and environmental factors may interrupt the adaptation process at any time throughout the life cycle. Dysfunction may occur when adaptation is impaired. Purposeful activity facilitates the adaptive process.
>
> Occupational therapy is based on the belief that purposeful activity (occupation), including its interpersonal and environmental components, may be used to prevent and mediate dysfunction, and to elicit maximum adaptation. Activity, as used by the Occupational Therapist, includes both an intrinsic and a therapeutic purpose. (116; p. 1)

Because this statement is relatively recent, no analyses or discussions of it are available in the literature. Further, the statement as published included no definition of terms or references. This may have been an oversight and further elaboration may be available in the future.

In the interim, to complement the "Philosophical Base" as presented above, five philosophical assumptions drawn from the literature of occupational therapy are offered for consideration (11,31,38,48,50,70,82, 103,105,128,135,145,146,151,160,169). These assumptions seem to be derived from those schools of philosophy that have been identified as pragmatic, existentialistic, and humanistic. All of these systems or schools of philosophy were predominant at the time of the profession's formal beginning. They continue to be held in high regard by many today. The philosophical assumptions are as follows.

1. *Each individual has the right to a meaningful existence; to an existence that allows one to be productive, to experience pleasure and joy, to love and be loved, and to live in safe, supportive, and comfortable surroundings.*

The idea of "meaningful existence" is important for several reasons. First, this assumption may be contrasted with one of the philosophical assumptions of the medical model: that the individual has a right to life. The kind of life is not taken into consideration. Traditionally, medicine has been concerned with the maintenance of life. Once life is maintained there is little concern for habilitation, rehabilitation, or the quality of life which is maintained. The right to life is considered paramount regardless of the wishes of the individual or the family or the needs of society. This is not to say that individual physicians are not concerned with quality of life; indeed, many physicians are. But such concern has not traditionally been part of the philosophical assumptions of medicine.

This assumption of the occupational therapy model implies—indeed, mandates—that once life is maintained the individual has a right to a meaningful existence. This right extends to the child who will never voluntarily lift its head, respond to another human being, or speak a word; to the adult who has lost control of defecation and urination, is wasted by malignant growths, or communicates only with obscenities. Each individual is considered to have the right to be treated as a unique and special person regardless of his current status or ability to be a productive member of the community.

Another reason why the idea of a meaningful existence is important is that it serves as the basis for two significant aspects of occupational therapy: (a) concern for the maintenance of function and (b) care of the chronically impaired individual. These aspects of occupational therapy are interrelated and complementary. Maintenance of function is the process of preserving and supporting an individual's current abilities to engage in interpersonal relationships and to manipulate the nonhuman environment. Concern for the care of individuals who are chronically impaired can be contrasted with concern for acute or temporary disability. Occupational therapists are concerned with the latter, but more than many other health professionals they are involved in the care of the chronically impaired. Whether these individuals reside in the community or in a sheltered environment, the occupational therapist helps them sustain a meaningful existence.

2. *Each individual is influenced by stage-specific maturation of the species, the social nature of the species, and the cognitive structure of the species.*

From this philosophical assumption occupational therapy has derived its special interest in the process of human growth and development. Theories relative to the maturation process are included in the theoretical foundation of occupational therapy; the chronological and developmental age of a client is taken into consideration in the evaluation and intervention processes.

Further elaboration may clarify this assumption. "Maturation" refers to the growth and change of an individual from conception until death. It refers to the entire life span rather than to only one particular portion, and has biological, sociological, and psychological dimensions. Biological maturation, perhaps the most predictable aspect of development in the sense of typical maturation, is also predictable in the sense of usual physical reactions to disease or injury. Biological maturation also appears to form the substratum for all other aspects of development. The sociological and psychological maturation of the individual is less predictable because of cultural differences. Usual patterns and the age at which specific skills are acquired vary among cultural groups. However, within the context of a culture there are fairly stable norms.

"The social nature of the species" refers to the individual's need for human interaction throughout the life span (34). As far as we know human beings have always lived in some group constellation. In addition to the early, relatively long period of dependency, there is an ongoing desire for human interaction. Moreover, it is fairly apparent that human interaction is essential for biological, sociological, and psychological maturation.

"The inherent cognitive structure of the species" refers not only to our seemingly greater intellectual capacity than other species but also to the way in which we use and process information. Human beings have an awareness of self; we are self-conscious. Because of our cognitive sophistication we have more choices than other animals. Conversely, we are subject to more psychological stress. This stress may lead to involvement in a variety of creative endeavors or it may lead to guilt, anxiety, depression, and the like. In addition, our cognitive structure influences our shared ability to use language, to conceptualize and identify relationships among events, to contemplate the future. What is of importance here is the commonality of our cognitive processes. We understand the symbolic meaning of a circle; "defense mechanisms" are a universal phenomenon; although difficult at times, one language can be translated into another.

Finally, this assumption is a statement about the shared nature of each human being. It is a statement of a belief that our inherent biological composition, dependence on social interaction, and cognitive organization define both our potentials and limitations.

3. *Each individual has the right to seek his or her potential through personal choice within the context of some social constraints.*

This philosophical assumption is reflected in the code of ethics of occupational therapy and in the profession's commitment to the possibility for individual growth and change. Again, clarification of terms used in this assumption may be useful. Given an individual's inherent capacities, "potential" refers to what an individual can do regardless of various limitations. A disability of one type or another need not be a limiting factor in being productive and finding satisfaction in life.

"Personal choice" refers to the right of an individual to decide to what degree, how, and in what way he will seek to reach his potential. Thus the individual has the option to engage in or refuse any type of evaluation or intervention process. Occupational therapists are responsible for explaining the various consequences of not engaging in the habilitation or rehabilitation process and for designing methods of intervention that are stimulating for the client. But ultimately it is the client's right and privilege to determine how he wishes to live his life.

Occupational therapists often work with clients who appear unable to engage, with knowledge, in the types of choice outlined above. In such an interaction, the therapist may continue to discuss and demonstrate the consequences of participation and nonparticipation in the intervention process. The therapist may also enlist the aid of other team members, family, and friends. However, the choice is finally that of the client.

The individual's right in this area has been described as limited "within some social constraints." Unless one decides to become a hermit, an individual is part of a community of others. Some behaviors are not tolerated by a particular community. The individual has the choice of acknowledging the constraints of a particular society, moving into another society, or accepting the consequences of engaging in behavior considered deviant by the society. Again there is the matter of individual choice. However, the society in which an individual lives also has rights that must be respected.

4. *Each individual is able to reach his or her potential only through purposeful interaction with the human and nonhuman environments.*

This philosophical assumption emphasizes the belief that learning is facilitated through doing, through interaction in concrete, immediate situations. Experiences that deal purely with the abstract or hypothetical are considered to be less conducive to integrated learning. This belief is not related to any particular theory of learning. Thus it is an assumption and not a part of occupational therapy's theoretical foundation.

The term *purposeful* relative to interaction or activity has been defined in a variety of ways. The Fidlers' (46; p. 305) definition is perhaps one of the most succinct. Purposeful activities are doing processes directed toward a planned or hypothesized end result. They provide an opportunity for "investigating, trying out and gaining evidence of one's capacities for experiencing, responding, managing, creating and controlling." In contrast, random activities are undirected and without a predetermined goal. Purposeful activities or interactions are one of the legitimate tools of occupational therapy. They are discussed in greater detail in Chapter 11.

This philosophical assumption also emphasizes the importance of both the human and nonhuman environments in the practice of occupational therapy. The term *activity* in the literature of the profession has in some periods been used to identify an individual's interaction primarily with the nonhuman environment. In other periods the importance of the interpersonal relationship between therapist and client has been stressed. The knowledge, skills, and attitudes acquired through purposeful interaction with the environment, in its totality, are the essence of the occupational therapy process.

5. *Each individual has inherent needs for work, play, and rest which must be satisfied in a relatively equal balance.*

This philosophical assumption became part of the occupational therapy model seemingly from its inception. Meyer and Slagle, early contributors to the profession, both believed that an optimal balance between work, play, and rest was a major factor in the restoration of function and the promotion of health. This assumption is reflected in the profession's theoretical foundation and domain of concern.

The philosophical assumptions of occupational therapy have been stated in a variety of ways throughout the profession's development. The differences, however, appear to be ones of semantics rather than substance. In actuality, there has been considerable consistency in the philosophical assumptions from the formal beginning of the profession.

6/ *Ethical Code of Occupational Therapy*

The ethical code of a profession serves as a guide for practitioners in determining what is moral behavior relative to clients and colleagues. In addition, it serves as a contract with the society to which the profession is responsible (7,24,41,58,138,159).

The code of ethics of occupational therapy, similar to that of many other health professions, was, in part, derived from the Hippocratic Oath. In order to appreciate the difference between the Hippocratic Oath and the occupational therapy code of ethics, the Oath is presented here.

> I swear by Apollo Physician, by Asclepius, by Health, by Panacea, and by all the gods and goddesses, making them my witnesses, that I will carry out, according to my ability and judgement, this oath and this indenture. To hold my teacher in this art equal to my own parents; to make him partner in my livelihood; when he is in need of money to share mine with him; to consider his family as my own brothers, and to teach them this art, if they want to learn it, without fee or indenture; to impart precept, oral instruction, and all other instruction to my own sons, the sons of my teacher, and to indentured pupils who have taken the physicians oath, but to nobody else. I will use treatment to help the sick according to my ability and judgement, but never with a view to injury and wrongdoing. Neither will I administer a poison to anybody when asked to do so, nor will I suggest such a course. Similarly I will not give a woman a pessary to cause abortion. But I will keep pure and holy both my life and my art. I will not use the knife, not ever, verily, on sufferers from stone, but I will give place to such as are craftsmen therein. Into whatsoever houses I enter, I will enter to help the sick, and I will abstain from all intentional wrongdoing and harm, especially from abusing the bodies of man or woman, bond or free. And whatsoever I shall see or hear in the course of my profession, as well as outside my profession in my intercourse with men, if it be what should not be published abroad, I will never divulge, holding such things to be holy secrets. Now if I carry out this oath, and break it not, may I gain forever reputation among all men for my life and for my art; but if I transgress it and forswear myself, may the opposite befall me. (159; p. 45)

The Hippocratic Oath covers many issues of concern to both the health professional and society. However, some issues are not addressed (24), such as the right of the patient to be an active participant in making choices about his treatment. Concomitant with that right is the patient's right to have sufficient information to make informed decisions. The Oath assumes that the patient, practitioner, and society have similar or congruent values, which in a pluralistic society is not always the case. The continuing controversy regarding the use of extraordinary means to sustain or prolong life and the issue of abortion are illustrative of differing values. The Oath is primarily centered on the individual and does not deal with the rights of society versus the rights of the individual. For example, does society have the right to sterilize individuals who are severely mentally retarded? The Hippocratic Oath does not deal with practitioner responsibility for the client when this responsibility is shared with other members of the health team and an institution. The question of whether the team as a whole and the institution are responsible or if the assigned leader of the team alone is responsible is not addressed. This also brings up the issue of whether responsibility is or should be delegated by a physician or shared by the health team.

The earliest published ethical code for occupational therapy is the "Pledge and Creed for Occupational Therapists:"

> Reverently and earnestly do I pledge my whole-hearted service in aiding those crippled in mind and body.
> To this end that my work for the sick may be successful, I will ever strive for greater knowledge, skill and understanding in the discharge of my duties in whatsoever position I may find myself.
> I solemnly declare that I will hold and keep inviolate whatever I may learn of the lives of the sick.
> I acknowledge the dignity of the cure of disease and the safeguarding of health in which no act is menial or inglorious.
> I will walk in upright faithfulness and obedience to those under whose guidance I am to work, and I pray for patience, kindliness and strength in the holy ministry to broken minds and bodies. (159; p. 45)

Carlotta Wells (159; p. 45) provides an excellent critique of the "Pledge and Creed" and a rationale for the major revisions that have been made. She states:

> The Pledge and Creed is in conflict with some laws and customs of today. Statements such as "broken minds and bodies" and "crippled in mind and body" do not fit modern descriptions of those who receive our services. Similarly, "Hold

and keep inviolate whatever I may learn of the lives of the sick" may not be in accord with present day ideas on the use of information about the patient to further his care. Although it indicates a helping attitude, "no act is menial or inglorious" may not be in accord with the need for personnel to function at their highest skill and, on the other hand, may contribute to the waste of personnel time, a significant expense to the institution. "I will walk in upright faithfulness and obedience to those under whose guidance I am to work" may prompt one unwittingly to commit an illegal act. The law expects one to be competent and to function within this competence, which may require an individual to refuse to follow an order known to be wrong or for which the individual is not qualified.

In 1976 the American Occupational Therapy Association appointed a Task Force on Ethics to formulate a revised code of ethics for the profession. The Task Force submitted a final draft of their work to the American Occupational Therapy Assocation's Representative Assembly, May 1977. The report was accepted and adopted. The report, entitled the "Principles of Occupational Therapy Ethics," is presented below in full:

Principles of Occupational Therapy Ethics

Preamble:

This Association and its component members are committed to furthering man's ability to function fully within his total environment. To this end the occupational therapist renders service to clients in all stages of health and illness, to institutions, other professionals, colleagues, students and to the general public.

In furthering this commitment the American Occupational Therapy Association has established the Principles of Occupational Therapy Ethics. It is intended that they be used by all occupational therapy personnel, including practitioners in all settings, administrators, educators, and students. These principles should be reflected in and supported by licensing laws, regulations, consultation, planning and teaching. They are intended to be action oriented, guiding and preventive rather than negative or merely disciplinary. However, it is intended that these principles are only for internal use by the American Occupational Therapy Association as a guide to appropriate conduct of its members, and it is not intended as a definition for patients or clients of a standard of care expected in any community. Professional maturity will be demonstrated in applying these basic principles while exercising the large measure of freedom which they provide and which is essential to responsible and creative occupational therapy service. For the purpose of continuity the following definitions will support information in this document: Occupational therapist includes registered occupational therapists, certified occupational therapy assistants, occupational therapy students. Clients include patients and those to whom occupational therapy services are delivered.

I—Related to the Recipient of Service

The occupational therapist demonstrates a beneficent concern for the recipient of services and maintains a goal-directed relationship with the recipient which furthers the objectives for which it is established. Services are evaluated against objectives and accountability is maintained therefore. Respect shall be shown for the recipients' rights and the occupational therapist will preserve the confidence of the patient relationship.

II—Related to Competence

The occupational therapist shall actively maintain and improve one's professional competence, represent it accurately, and function within its perimeters.

III—Related to Records, Reports, Grades and Recommendations

The occupational therapist shall conform to local, state and federal laws and regulations and regulations applicable to records and reports. The occupational therapist abides by the employing institution's rules. Objective data shall govern subjective data in evaluations, grades, recommendations, records and reports.

IV—Related to Intra-professional Colleagues

The occupational therapist shall function with discretion and integrity in relations with other members of the profession and shall be concerned with the quality of their services. Upon becoming aware of objective evidence of a breach of ethics or substandard service, the occupational therapist shall take action according to established procedure.

V—Related to Other Personnel

The occupational therapist shall function with discretion and integrity in relations with personnel and cooperate with them as may be appropriate. Similarly, the occupational therapist expects others to demonstrate a high level of competence. Upon becoming aware of objective evidence of a breach of ethics or substandard service, the occupational therapist shall take action according to established procedure.

VI—Related to Employers and Payers

The occupational therapist shall render service with discretion and integrity and shall protect the property and property rights of the employers and payers.

VII—Related to Education

The occupational therapist implements a commitment to the education of society and the consumer of health services as well as to the education of health personnel on matters of health which are within the purview of occupational therapy.

VIII—Related to Evaluation and Research

The occupational therapist shall accept responsibility for evaluating, developing and refining service and the body of knowledge and skills which underlie the education and practice of occupational therapy and at all times protect the rights of subjects, clients, institutions and collaborators. The work of others shall be acknowledged.

IX—Related to the Profession

The occupational therapist shall be responsible for gaining information and understanding of the principles, policies and standards of the profession. The occupational therapist functions as a representative of the profession.

X—Related to Law and Regulations
The occupational therapist shall seek to acquire information about applicable local, state, federal and institutional rules and shall function accordingly thereto.

XI—Related to Misconduct
The occupational therapist shall not appear to act with impropriety nor engage in illegal conduct involving moral turpitude and will not circumvent the principles of occupational therapy ethics through actions of another.

XII—Related to Bioethical Issues and Problems of Society
The occupational therapist seeks information about the major health problems and issues to learn their implications for occupational therapy and for one's own services. (7; p. E-11)

Although far superior to both the Hippocratic Oath and the "Pledge and Creed for Occupational Therapists," the "Principles of Occupational Therapy Ethics" described above has some deficits.

Principle I states that the occupational therapist "will preserve the confidence of the patient relationship." This statement may be misleading for those therapists who are members of a team. Information provided by the client must be shared with other team members. If one or more team members have an exclusive, confidential relationship with a client, the purpose and function of a team are weakened. In addition, the client has a right to know that information given to one team member will be shared with other team members.

Principle VII is concerned with the responsibility of occupational therapists to educate others "on matters of health which are within the purview of occupational therapy." However, no mention is made of the responsibility of occupational therapists to educate students of occupational therapy. Adequate education of students who will soon become colleagues in practice is paramount for the continuation and growth of any profession.

Principle VIII emphasizes the importance of research. However, there is no mention of the occupational therapist's responsibility to publish and make use of research findings. This may have been assumed by the writers of the document. But a clear statement may highlight the importance of this area of professional responsibility.

Principle IX focuses on the responsibility of the occupational therapist to acquire "information and understanding of the principles, policies and standards of the profession." What the Principle does not describe is the therapist's responsibility for *participation* in developing the principles, policies, and standards of the profession. The obligation of the therapist to be involved in local, state, and the national organization is not mentioned. Within these organizations principles, policies, and standards are formulated.

Finally, Principle XII, which is concerned with the bioethical issues and problems of society, provides minimal guidelines for the practitioner (58). Even the most current issues such as abortion, the use of extraordinary means to prolong life, and euthanasia are not addressed.

In addition to the above, the "Principles of Occupational Therapy Ethics" do not attempt to deal with the following significant issues:

1. The idea of a reasonable fee for service;
2. The therapist's responsibility for not following an order or prescription that the therapist believes would be harmful to a client's well-being;
3. The need to provide sufficient information to enable the client or those responsible for the client to make informed decisions regarding evaluation and intervention;
4. The conflict which may arise between the rights of the client and the rights of society;
5. The question of who is ultimately responsible to the client when evaluation and intervention take place within the context of a team and/or an institution.

In time, the areas of practice not mentioned in the "Principles of Occupational Therapy Ethics" are likely to be addressed. This code of ethics is relatively new and thus is likely to be subject to revisions in the future. No profession has a code of ethics that provides guidelines for every aspect of practice. The issues encountered in practice change far more rapidly than a profession's code of ethics. In this time lapse, practitioners must use their own personal ethical system as a guide for day-to-day interaction with clients and colleagues.

This chapter opened with a presentation of the Hippocratic Oath. The ethical code of medicine of today is much more comprehensive and detailed. Yet the Hippocratic Oath continues to influence physicians, members of other health professions, and their clients. An oath or pledge has an emotional impact not found in the rather dry statement of ethical principles. Thus an oath for occupational therapists, formulated by the author, is presented below. It is presented, hopefully, in the spirit of the Hippocratic Oath with its reverence for the responsibilities and privileges of practice, teaching, and scholarly pursuits:

As an occupational therapist I will: revere the quality of life above life itself; assist all who request my help according to my ability and judgement; provide sufficient information to enable my client or those responsible for my client to make informed decisions regarding intervention; respect my client's right to self-determination; protect the confidence of my client, sharing only with those others who are immediately involved with my client's care; be goal directed and objective in my evaluation and intervention; follow only those recommendations that I judge as being beneficial to my client; maintain my competence and represent that competence accurately; accept my own limitations and when indicated seek the assistance of those with different or greater knowledge and skill; ask only a reasonable fee for service; take responsibility for participating in formulating the policies and standards of my profession; build upon the knowledge and skills of those who have come before me, giving full recognition to their contributions; share my knowledge and skills with those who will follow through publication and teaching; respect my colleagues to the extent that they deserve my respect; condemn those colleagues who are incompetent or unethical in practice; be accountable for all my decisions and actions.

To the members of my profession and the society to which I am responsible and serve, I make this pledge with full understanding of the actions required by this oath.

7 / Theoretical Foundation of Occupational Therapy

The theoretical foundation of a profession is a statement of selected theories from various fields of inquiry which serve as the scientific bases for practice (71,147). Selected theories from the biological sciences, psychology, sociology, the arts, and medicine and theories generated through the practice of occupational therapy form the theoretical foundation of occupational therapy (128).

In contrast, the theoretical foundation of medicine is derived primarily from the biological sciences. Emphasis is on the cause and alteration of disease processes and the repair of injury. The theories developed by the various psychoanalytic and ego psychology schools of thought are part of the theoretical base of psychiatry but only tangential to the theoretical foundation of medicine as a whole. The theoretical foundation of the medical model is primarily oriented to defining illness and how to assist an individual to move from a state of illness to a state of not being ill.

The theoretical foundation of occupational therapy is different and far broader. Occupational therapy is concerned with the body, mind, and environment of the individual. These three aspects of the individual are considered to be inseparable. Thus evaluation and intervention involve the individual as a totality regardless of which areas of function are identified as being deficient. For example, a 6-year-old child born with cardiac insufficiency may have corrective surgery. After surgery the occupational therapist's primary concern is likely to be increasing strength and endurance. However, the occupational therapist is also concerned with secondary deficits consequential to cardiac insufficiency. Intervention, therefore, might also be directed to the development of age-appropriate social skills, independence in self-care, and learning how to enjoy the typical active games of childhood.

An in-depth description of the theoretical foundation of occupational therapy is not possible in a text of this nature. Thus the following outline indicates only broad areas of theories that form the substratum for practice (6,65).

AREAS OF THEORY

Biological Sciences

Anatomy; physiology; neuroanatomy; neurophysiology; biomechanics; development and maturation of the neuromuscular, skeletal, sensory, and endocrine systems; the various relationships between the biological systems; conservation of physical energy.

Psychology

Development and maintenance of sensory integrative and cognitive processes, learning, personality development, measurement and testing, psychoanalytic theory, object relations, ego psychology, psychodynamics, symbolism, psychosocial and psychosexual development, the psychological impact of stress, the psychological aspects of various life stages, the psychological components of disability and chronic illness, psychological needs, the counseling process, industrial psychology, the significance of play and recreation in the life cycle.

Sociology

The dynamics of primary and secondary groups; the dynamics of the family; the process of child rearing; varieties of life styles; development of morality and a system of values; the socialization process and social deviancy; the structure and process of groups that can be directed toward facilitating growth, satisfying needs, and maintaining function; human relations, communication theory, industrial sociology relative to management, supervision and administration; the nature of work; occupational choice, career change, and various career patterns; the structure and dynamics of a community; community resources; the nature of various social systems; cultural differences in life styles, values, and norms; role theory.

The Arts

Fine, applied, industrial, and manual arts; dance; music; literature.

Medicine

The sequelae of disease, trauma, genetic deficits, and stress; positive and negative factors that influence intervention relative to sequelae, course, and prognosis of various diagnostic categories; general principles of rehabilitation.

Occupational Therapy

The nature of the nonhuman environment as it influences development and the alteration of dysfunction; the nature and use of purposeful activities to develop, maintain, and facilitate function; the dynamics and processes of activity groups; the design and fabrication of functional aids and adaptive equipment and the impact of these aids and equipment on the ability of the individual to function comfortably in his selected life style; the various means whereby the function and dysfunction of concern to the occupational therapist are identified; the means by which dysfunction is prevented, minimized, or eliminated; the use of functional capacities to minimize deficits in other areas of function (6,48,65,82,91,101,129,143,154).

CHANGES IN THEORY

The theoretical foundation of occupational therapy, as with the theoretical foundation of all professions, changes over time as new phenomena are studied, new theories developed, and older theories further verified or refuted. The theoretical foundation of occupational therapy is considerable. There is, however, a difference in the degree to which the various theories that comprise the theoretical foundation of occupational therapy have been verified through empirical research.

8 / Domain of Concern of Occupational Therapy

The domain of concern of a profession is those areas of human experience in which practitioners of the profession offer assistance to others. It is essentially a statement of what the profession believes to be its area of expertise (53,107).

The domain of concern of medicine is pathological conditions resulting from disease, trauma, or genetic deficit. It is concerned with what is commonly defined as illness or physical injury by a particular society. Until recently, the domain of concern of medicine has been oriented primarily to the treatment of acute conditions. Now there is additional emphasis on chronic conditions such as circulatory and respiratory problems. This change appears to be due to the control of many contagious diseases, the availability of antibiotics, and an increase in the average age of the population.

The domain of concern of occupational therapy is here described as consisting of performance components within the context of age, occupational performance, and an individual's environment (65,69,70,78,91, 92,111,124,127,128,132,145,154). Figure 2 is an attempt to illustrate in graphic form the domain of concern of occupational therapy and the relationship among its component parts.

This diagram may need some explanation and definition of terms. Performance components are here considered to be the core of the occupational therapy domain of concern. *Core* refers to the primary or first area of consideration in the evaluation and intervention process. The performance components described below are broadly defined. They are defined in a more specific and detailed manner in the profession's various frames of reference.

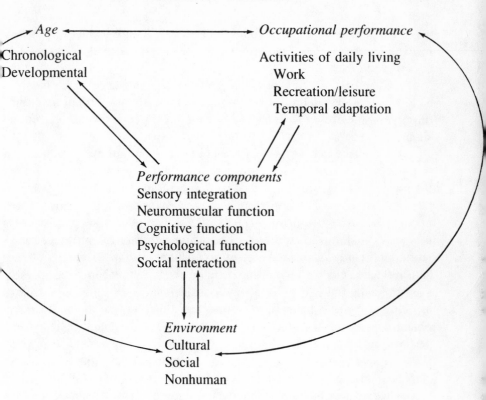

FIG. 2. Domain of concern for occupational therapy.

Sensory integration is the ability to receive, differentiate, perceive, and use sensory stimuli for planned interaction with one's external environment.

Neuromuscular function is the ability to use one's body to act effectively relative to the environment. This includes reflex integration, coordination, range of motion, strength, and endurance.

Cognitive function is the ability to (a) learn at a rate comparable to one's peers in chronological age; (b) comprehend one's past, present, and anticipated future environment relative to time, place, and significant individuals; (c) conceptualize, establish abstract relationships, and solve problems within the logical system of one's culture.

Psychological function is the ability to process information from past events and information currently available from the environment in such a way as to perceive oneself and others realistically. It also includes the ability to experience, identify, and express emotions in a manner acceptable to oneself and others.

Social interaction refers to that area of human experience which involves a close, sustained relationship with other individuals; friendship, love, nurturing; and the ability to engage in a variety of groups of meaningful and significant others.

Age, occupational performance, and environment are the parameters of occupational therapy's domain of concern. *Parameters* here refers to both the boundary of occupational therapy's domain of concern and the importance of age, occupational performance, and environment in evaluation and intervention. The boundary of occupational therapy's domain of concern designates the limits of expertise of occupational therapists. But, and perhaps more importantly, the parameters of occupational therapy's domain of concern influence evaluation and intervention. For example, in assessing sensory integration, the therapist always considers the age of the individual; in assisting a client to increase neuromuscular function, the therapist always remains aware of what activities of daily living the client can possibly perform independently in the future; in assisting an individual to develop skills in social interaction, the therapist attempts to identify what is acceptable and expected social behavior in the client's cultural group.

The parameters of the occupational therapy domain of concern may be clarified by a few more definitions.

AGE

Chronological age is the number of days, months, and years an individual has lived since the day of birth.

Developmental age refers to the level of function in performance components in comparison to the approximate age-specific norms of the individual's cultural group. Developmental age is not necessarily related to chronological age.

OCCUPATIONAL PERFORMANCE

Activities of daily living are all those activities one must engage in or accomplish to be able to participate with comfort in other facets of life.

These activities may be subdivided into self-care, communication, and travel. Self-care includes such areas as maintaining proper hygiene, grooming, dressing, eating, preparing meals, and handling money. Communication refers to such things as the ability to engage in conversation with another individual, use the telephone, write personal and business letters, and complete a variety of forms. Travel refers to the ability to use public transportation; read and follow a bus, subway, or road map; drive a car; get a taxi; or find information as to how to arrive at a given destination.

Work is an individual's major occupation. It includes remunerative employment, paramount avocational pursuits, the responsibilities of a homemaker, the process of parenting, the activities of a student relative to school work, and the play of a child. The latter is often not thought of as work. However, through play a child develops cognitive and motor skills and learns about himself, other people, and society. Mastery of the area of work requires certain knowledge and skills. These are often referred to as "work habits." Some examples of work habits are the ability to get to work on time, dress appropriately, accept direction from a work supervisor or teacher, get along with one's co-workers, and take responsibility for assigned tasks. Other more specific knowledge and skills are required for a particular job, but these specialized tasks are not considered to be in the domain of concern of occupational therapy.

Recreation/leisure refers to engaging in activities for the sake of amusement, relaxation, or self-actualization. There are two aspects to recreation. One involves those things a person does for fun. Depending on the individual, this might include such things as reading a novel, playing tennis, taking care of a garden, or going to a party. The other aspect of recreation involves participating in community activities, for example, doing volunteer work in a nursing home, coaching a girls' softball team, participating in local political organizations, or tutoring students.

Temporal adaptation is first the ability to organize one's time in order to fulfill various role responsibilities. Most individuals have several roles. For example, one may be a mother, lover, lawyer, friend, and chairperson of a tenant association. The other aspect of temporal adaptation is the ability to satisfy one's multiple needs in a manner that promotes physical and psychological health. Human needs have been described in a variety of ways and are discussed in more detail in Chapter 9. Suffice it to say here that individuals need to work, play, and rest. Temporal adaptation refers to one's ability to satisfy these needs in a relatively equal manner.

ENVIRONMENT

Environment, the third part of the parameters of occupational therapy's domain of concern, includes the individual's cultural, social, and nonhuman environment.

Cultural environment refers to a client's past, present, and anticipated future involvement in a cultural system. A cultural system consists of social structures, values, norms, and expectations accepted and shared by a group of people. The individual's attitudes about and degree of involvement in the evaluation and intervention process are often strongly influenced by membership in past and present cultural systems. The therapist's understanding and appreciation of the client's cultural background greatly increases the possibility of successful intervention. In addition, if the client's anticipated future cultural environment is likely to be different from past cultural environments, the therapist must take this into consideration in the intervention process. For example, in assisting a Cuban refugee to develop various performance components, the therapist would also be concerned with the client's knowledge of and adjustment to a new cultural environment.

Social environment refers to the matrix of people with whom the client is presently related and to those people she or he will need to relate to in the future. These people may be family, friends, co-workers, and other significant individuals. The therapist is concerned about the client's feelings and typical patterns of interaction with these individuals. In addition, the therapist is concerned about the expectations of and degree of support available from the social environment. Many clients need to use a variety of unfamiliar community resources in order to maintain function and live comfortably within the community. Such resources may include a visiting nurse, food stamps, or recreational facilities. The client often needs to learn about these resources and how to relate to the various individuals who serve as the gatekeeper for these resources.

The *nonhuman environment* in the context of occupational therapy's domain of concern refers to the physical environment in which the individual lives or is likely to live in the future. This includes such things as possible architectural barriers that may impede the mobility of the physically disabled individual; the complexity of the environment which may cause difficulty for the cognitively impaired individual; ambience; the degree of physical safety; and the opportunity to be surrounded by nonhuman objects that have personal meaning to the individual.

With this final definition of the components of occupational therapy's domain of concern, the reader is referred to Fig. 2. The arrows connecting all of the parts of the domain of concern may need some further elaboration. In general, the arrows are meant to indicate the interrelationship of all parts of the domain of concern. Thus evaluation and intervention relative to performance components always take into consideration the client's age, current level of skill in the various areas of occupational performance, and future possible levels of skill in these areas and the client's past, present, and future expected environment. Thus, in evaluation and designing a plan for intervention in the area of cognitive function, for example, the therapist needs to know the age of the client, something about the client's recreational and work interests, and the values of the individual's cultural group.

In addition, knowledge of age and culture and social group membership will help the therapist to determine whether the client's functioning in the area of occupational performance is within the range of what is considered to be acceptable limits. In illustration, in some cultural groups or families an 11-year-old boy is expected to make his bed every morning and get ready for school independently, whereas in other cultural groups or families such behavior is not expected. Knowledge of a client's age, past engagement in the various areas of occupational performance, and past and future expected environment assists the therapist in designing plans for intervention that are most likely to provide a firm groundwork for the client's successful return to full participation in the life of the community.

As in the definitions of performance components, there is considerable overlap among the various aspects of occupational performance and between cultural and social environments. And many aspects of these parameters of the domain of concern are closely related to performance components. Although at times it is necessary to divide to understand, one of the major assets of the occupational therapy domain of concern is its interrelatedness of parts. Just as in a mosaic stained glass window, each piece is important but the parts together give us an appreciation of the whole.

9/ The Nature of and Principles for Sequencing the Various Aspects of Practice of Occupational Therapy

The nature of practice is essentially a definition of the various aspects of practice. Principles for sequencing the various aspects of practice refers to the way in which a profession identifies problems and then solves them (9,30,59,107,136,137,155).

To return once again to the medical model for illustrative purposes, the practice of medicine involves gaining information regarding signs and symptoms; determining cause, pathological processes, or both; ensuring prevention or instituting treatment; and understanding the typical course, prognosis, and sequelae of disease, injury, or deficits. For the reader unfamiliar with this terminology the following definitions might be useful:

A *sign* is an objective indicator of illness such as an elevated body temperature, fainting, or swelling of a body part. *Symptoms* are subjective phenomena that arise from and accompany a particular disease or disorder. Some examples of symptoms are headaches, nausea, chronic weakness, and lassitude. *Cause* is the event, circumstance, or agent that leads to disease or injury. *Disease* is a condition of the organism such that a type of cell or a structure is prevented from performing its usual function. *Pathology*, the study of diseases, refers to diseased, disordered, or abnormal conditions of the organism. *Prevention* is the process of eliminating causal factors prior to their possible negative impact on the human organism. Classic examples of prevention are the Salk vaccine for poliomyelitis and monitoring the level of exposure to radiation of individuals working with radioactive materials. *Treatment* is the process of minimizing or eliminating a pathological condition and, if possible, is directed toward the cause of the pathological condition. If this is not possible, treatment is directed toward minimizing the signs and symptoms of the pathological condition. For example, the cause of the common cold is unknown. Thus treatment is oriented to minimizing signs and symptoms. The common cold is treated with aspirin, bed rest, and sympathy.

Course refers to the typical progression or regression of a pathological condition and the stages inherent in the process. For example, the course of events relative to a bout with stomach flu is relatively familiar to all of us. *Prognosis* is a prediction of the duration and outcome of a pathological condition. In simple language, is one going to get better or worse. Finally, *sequelae* are the abnormal conditions resulting from a disease process, trauma, or genetic deficit. For example, common sequelae of a cerebral vascular accident (stroke) are motor weakness and diminished sensation on one side of the body.

In regard to principles for sequencing the various aspects of practice, the medical model identifies prevention as primary. Although prevention of disease, injury, or deficits is considered to be the first phase of medical practice, it is only a small part of most physicians' daily interaction with patients. The typical sequence of medical practice starts with diagnoses based on the client's signs and symptoms. Diagnosis is the process of identifying and labeling a particular disease process or injury. Once a diagnosis is made, the physician selects various legitimate tools and initiates treatment. Treatment is directed toward minimizing or eliminating the effects of causal factors or disease processes or diminishing the discomfort of signs and symptoms. In addition, treatment is guided by the physician's knowledge of the usual course, prognosis, and sequelae of the client's condition.

With this brief outline of the aspects of practice of the medical model, the nature of the various aspects of the practice of occupational therapy will be described. The practice of occupational therapy is concerned with identifying areas of function and dysfunction through the observation of specified behaviors. If it is determined that an individual is in a state of dysfunction in some particular area, he or she is invited and encouraged to participate in the occupational therapy intervention process. The author apologizes for another rather lengthy series of definitions which follow.

Function is the ability to engage comfortably at an age-appropriate level in performance components and the areas of occupational performance within the context of one's cultural, social, and nonhuman environment. *Dysfunction* is the inability to engage comfortably at an age-appropriate level in performance components or the areas of occupational performance within the context of one's cultural, social, and nonhuman environment. Dysfunction may be due to sequelae arising from disease, injury, or deficit. Thus the occupational therapist, unlike the physician, is not concerned with cause or pathological process, but rather with the consequence of causal factors or pathological processes. Dysfunction may be the loss of a particular skill or the lack of development of a particular skill in the usual course of maturation. Intervention in the former area is often referred to as rehabilitation, whereas intervention in the latter is referred to as habilitation (108).

Behaviors indicative of function and dysfunction are those behaviors that provide evidence for or indicate whether an individual is competent in the performance components and the areas of occupational performance relative to age and the individual's cultural, social, and nonhuman environment. These behaviors are outlined in detail in the various frames of reference of occupational therapy. Evaluation procedures are based on knowledge of behaviors indicative of function and dysfunction. Evaluation, briefly stated, is a collaborative process between client, therapist, and significant others to determine whether an individual is in need of or could benefit from occupational therapy intervention (11,16,47,65,80,101,108,154). Evaluation is defined more specifically after a discussion of the various types of occupational therapy intervention.

The *intervention process* involves a collaborative effort by client and therapist directed toward goals they have previously established. For the sake of clarity and specificity, intervention can be subdivided into five types: meeting health needs, prevention, the change process, maintenance, and management (1).

Meeting health needs is the process of satisfying or fulfilling inherent human needs so that an individual may experience a sense of physical, psychological, and social well-being (47,101). These needs are considered to be shared by all individuals regardless of their current state of health. Health needs may be differentiated from those needs that arise from the consequence of physical or psychosocial dysfunction. Thus, for example, the need for love and acceptance is considered to be a health need. Extreme psychological dependency of an adult is not considered to be a health need. The latter is evidence of dysfunction and is dealt with in the change process. Briefly, health needs are described as:

Psycho-physical: The need for adequate and attractive food, clothing and shelter; and for an optimal amount of sensory stimuli, gross motor activity and rest.

Security: The need for an environment characterized by a shared reality in which the majority of persons in the environment are in agreement regarding the nature of objects and the appropriate response to object, predictable responses from others, known expectations regarding appropriate behavior, relatively consistent ordering of events, recognition of the individual's right to need satisfaction, some degree of change as a consequence of the individual's actions, a manageable number of unknowns, and freedom from physical harm.

Love and acceptance: The need for positive response to one's unique being, as opposed to doing.

Group association: The need for regular and intimate interaction with an aggregate of others who share common interests and goals.

Esteem: The need for an opportunity to be a contributing member of a social system, and for recognition of and positive response to one's contributions.

Sexual: The need for recognition of one's sexual nature, association with both sexes, and release or sublimation of sexually induced tensions.

Developmental: The need for objects and interactions that are believed to promote acquisition of skills necessary for mature and gratifying interaction in the environment.

Pleasure: The need to engage in activities that the individual perceives as enjoyable in and of themselves.

This is, of course, only one way health needs may be categorized. Other systems may be preferred depending upon one's work setting, theoretical orientation, and world view. A specific way of conceptualizing health needs is not as important as grasping their nature and differentiating them from pathological needs. (101; pp. 14–15)

A client is sometimes not able to satisfy health needs without assistance. This may be due to dysfunction or the client's current environment. Current environment here refers to either an institutional setting or the community. Many institutions are not conducive to need satisfaction; many communities do not provide sufficient resources for the satisfaction of health needs for many of its members.

The responsibility for meeting health needs is not occupational therapists' alone but rather is shared with other members of the health team, clients, and community members. Two examples of programs designed to meet health needs are (a) helping clients and community members to organize various social and cultural activities for adults who are mentally retarded; (b) working with clients and other members of the health team to make clients' living quarters in an institution more attractive and comfortable.

In addition to humanitarian reasons, assisting clients to meet health needs is important because clients concerned primarily with need satisfaction are less likely to participate in other areas of intervention. The difference between meeting health needs and the change process will be discussed after the change process has been defined.

Prevention is the process of facilitating the development of skills in possible areas of dysfunction and promoting skills in areas of function (40,49,50,56,71,72,160). As used in this text, prevention refers to intervention prior to any evidence of dysfunction. Thus prevention defined here is similar to the idea of prevention as discussed in relationship to the medical model. The difference between the two is not in the idea itself but rather in the dissimilarity in the professions' domains of concern. For example, physicians are concerned with preventing rubella. Occupational therapists are not involved in implementing prevention in this area. Conversely, occupational therapists are concerned with the prevention of possible deterioration of social skills of individuals who are isolated from interaction in the community. Physicians are not usually involved in implementing prevention in this area.

Occupational therapists are involved in prevention in the areas of performance components and occupational performances. They are concerned with individuals or groups of individuals who are at risk for any number of reasons. Some of the major populations of concern are infants who are born prematurely, experienced severe birth trauma, or show some evidence of genetic deficits or developmental lag; individuals who live in an environment that does not satisfy health needs or are involved in a cultural/social environment that fosters antisocial behavior relative to the norms and values of the predominant culture; and individuals who experience a significant change in social roles, responsibilities, or mobility. Prevention may entail direct services to clients by the occupational therapist, or the therapist may serve as a consultant to other professionals who provide direct service. Finally, prevention may involve the education of parents, other family members, and the public.

The change process is concerned with the development or restoration of function to the highest possible level. The therapist and client anticipate and work toward significant change. The change process is directed toward enhancing the client's ability in the various areas of performance components and occupational performances (65,110,154). For example, the therapist may be concerned with increasing the client's physical coordination or in identifying and developing the skills necessary for participation in recreational activities the client enjoys.

In the change process, therapist and client are concerned with bringing about some predetermined planned change in the patient's repertoire of behavior. This is in contrast to meeting health needs. In the process of meeting health needs a client's behavior may change but the nature of the change is not predetermined or planned by the therapist or client. Another distinction between the change process and meeting health needs is the factor of time orientation. The change process is directed toward developing skills required for future interaction in the community. Meeting health needs is concerned with the client's current life situation.

Maintenance is the process of preserving and supporting an individual's current level of function (72,81,162). There are two somewhat different types of maintenance. One process involves maintaining function in one or more areas while attempting to alter dysfunction in other selected areas. For example, because of a cerebral vascular accident a client has moderately impaired sensory perception. In addition, the client has a history of a mild arthritic condition in the right hand and shoulder. As part of the change process, the therapist and client are involved with enhancing sensory perception. As part of maintenance the therapist is concerned with protecting and preserving function of the right hand and shoulder. In this example these two processes are likely to be concurrent in the daily interaction of therapist and client.

The other type of maintenance is entirely separate from the change process in relation to time. After the change process has ended, the therapist often continues to be concerned with maintenance of the degree of function that has been attained. Thus, for example, a home program to maintain strength in the upper extremities may be designed with a paraplegic client.

As mentioned previously, occupational therapists are oriented toward and committed to chronically disabled individuals. For many of these individuals further change is impossible and thus an unrealistic goal. However, these individuals often do need a variety of programs designed to maintain function. Occupational therapists are involved with, for example, clients who are able to participate in the community only marginally or who need the various services offered by a skilled nursing facility.

In the process of maintenance, the occupational therapist adjusts intervention in accordance with the clients' stability, progression, or regression in function. Although some clients' ability to function in various areas remains relatively stable for a long period of time, this is not true for other clients. Some diseases, such as neurological and collagen conditions, are characterized by alternating periods of exacerbation and remission. Maintenance in such cases involves closely monitoring the client's ability to function in various areas, and designing and redesigning programs to be in accord with the client's most current level of function.

Finally, *management* is the process of minimizing undesirable or disruptive behavior so the therapist can deal directly and effectively with areas of dysfunction (81). "Undesirable or disruptive behavior" may be behavior indicative of dysfunction. As such, it is not of direct concern in the change process, but is simply a manifestation of dysfunction. For example, in some frames of reference "hearing voices" that outline in graphic detail one's many limitations as a human being is indicative of an inaccurate self-concept. The change process based on such frames of reference would be directed toward developing a more accurate and adequate self-concept. The management part of intervention would be directed toward helping the client, at least for some period of time, to ignore the voices. While the client is attending to voices he or she is unlikely to engage in activities designed to correct self-concept. Management is concerned only with minimizing undesirable or disruptive behavior, not in changing that behavior *per se*. If the change process is successful, such behavior will gradually disappear as the individual acquires more functional skills in dealing with the self and the environment.

Undesirable and disruptive behavior may not be related to any particular area of dysfunction but be more general in nature. Recognizing dysfunction, electing to engage in a change process, or perhaps being in a strange environment is likely to cause anxiety, which may be manifest in a variety of ways. For example, a 13-year-old boy with multiple fractures may exhibit a facade of bravado and sophistication that is both unrelated to his real feelings and detrimental to engaging in the change process. A 3-year-old child huddled in the corner with tears in her eyes is not going to be a willing participant in an activity designed to enhance tactile discrimination. The therapist, then, must be concerned with those behaviors that arise out of anxiety. In dealing with such behavior, the therapist not only decreases anxiety but also increases the individual's capacity to participate in the change process.

For the sake of clarification, intervention is described above as having five distinct parts. As may be apparent to the reader, there is some overlapping or area of commonality among the five aspects of intervention. They have been separated here to describe the distinct differences. In the actual intervention process, the various aspects of intervention may blend one with the other. A note of caution: in this possible blending a wise therapist knows each part included in any particular plan for intervention.

Now that intervention has been described in some detail, evaluation can be defined more specifically: *evaluation* is the process of assessing whether an individual requires assistance in meeting health needs in his or her current environment, is in need of intervention directed toward prevention, is able to benefit from involvement in the change process, or is in need of a program of maintenance or management. Evaluation takes place prior to and periodically during the course of intervention. Evaluation is concerned with the current status of the individual. Intervention involves some modification of current status.

The second and related part of this component of the occupational therapy model is the sequence of the various aspects of practice (21,93,127,158). The following sequence of events appears to be fairly typical and is based on the definitions of terms in the preceding section.

Initial evaluation is directed toward determining the need for occupational therapy intervention and the type(s) of intervention required. Evaluation takes place periodically throughout the intervention process. After initial evaluation, if intervention is indicated, the therapist is first concerned with meeting health needs and prevention. Maintenance of current function is the next priority. If necessary, intervention is then directed toward management. This accomplished, the therapist focuses attention on the change process. In the change process, intervention is usually first directed toward correcting dysfunction in performance components. As a client becomes more skilled in performance components, more concentrated effort is directed toward occupational performance. For example, as neuromotor function increases, the therapist and client may spend an increasing amount of time in developing self-care skills. When the client cannot attain a sufficient level of function in one or more of the performance components, the therapist assists the client in developing substitute skills—those which serve as a means of compensating for lack of function in one or more of the performance components. For example, an individual unable to regain an adequate degree of sensory and motor function in one hand may be assisted in learning how to become competent in performing a number of activities with the use of only one hand. Finally, the therapist assists the client in identifying and planning the ways in which function will be maintained after intervention is terminated.

The typical sequence of practice outlined above is general in nature. The sequence may be altered because of the special needs of a particular client or the environment in which evaluation and intervention take place. An example of the first situation is the 7-year-old child who wants desperately to learn how to dress herself. She feels embarrassed and inadequate because she has not mastered the skill. Lack of such mastery appears to be due to a major deficit in sensory integration. However, because of this young client's concern, the therapist may begin by teaching this one skill concurrent with attempting to increase function in the more basic area of deficit (81). An example of the influence of environment on the sequence of practice is the realistic constraints of a facility that can offer only short-term care. In such a facility the therapist often can be concerned only with evaluation and meeting health needs, giving the change process and maintenance only minimal attention.

In summary, this chapter describes the nature of occupational therapy practice and the sequence of the various aspects of practice. This brief outline is presented only as an orientation; within the context of practice the richness and diversity of occupational therapy become apparent.

10/ *Legitimate Tools of Occupational Therapy*

Legitimate tools, the sixth and last component of a profession's model, are the permissible means by which the practitioners of a given profession fulfill their responsibility to society. Through using its tools a profession attempts to achieve its goals in meeting specific needs of a society.

Traditionally, the major legitimate tools of medicine have been drugs, surgical procedures, and conscious use of self. The reader is sufficiently aware of the nature of drugs and surgical procedures that no definition is needed. Conscious use of self is a tool occupational therapy shares with medicine and thus is defined in the discussion of that tool.

It appears from a review of the literature and practice that occupational therapy has six legitimate tools. These are the nonhuman environment, conscious use of self, teaching-learning process, purposeful activities, activity groups, and activity analysis and synthesis. A short description of these tools makes up the remainder of this chapter.

NONHUMAN ENVIRONMENT

The term *nonhuman environment* refers to all aspects of the environment that are not human. Occupational therapists view the nonhuman environment as an entity to be mastered, an aid to facilitate the performance of life tasks, and a vehicle for assisting in the development of sensory, cognitive, and motor skills and need-fulfilling intrapersonal and interpersonal relationships. Some examples of how an occupational therapist uses the nonhuman environment in the evaluation and intervention process are provided in Chapter 1. No further description is given here. Rather, this section focuses on the nature of the nonhuman environment primarily as it has been articulated by

Harold Searles (143). Three aspects of the nonhuman environment are discussed: (a) the way in which the nonhuman environment facilitates normal growth and development; (b) the nonhuman environment as a possible source of anxiety; and (c) the ways in which constructive interaction with the nonhuman environment can be impeded.

One of the first tasks of the infant is to differentiate between the self and the environment. Much has been written about the differentiation process relative to the human environment. For example, the child at some point distinguishes between herself and her mother. But in order to see the self as truly human one must also identify basic differences between what is human and what is not human. Through stimulation by the nonhuman environment and self-stimulation, the infant begins to perceive "the me versus the not me," or what is external to the self as opposed to internal to the self. Through interaction with various components of the nonhuman environment the child begins to identify characteristics unique to human beings. This latter process continues through life and, in some ways, is never really completed. An illustration of this is the tendency to attribute human feelings to favored pets or plants.

The nonhuman environment contributes to one's sense of security. It tends often to be more stable and predictable than the human environment. Periodic changes in the nonhuman environment do occur, but they are likely to be rhythmic. In addition, the nonhuman environment often offers a continuity of experience as one moves through time and space. For example, offering a visitor food and something to drink not only is something we were taught to do as children but is a custom common to most of the cultural groups we are likely to encounter in our adult life. The nonhuman environment provides a sense of security in a physical manner: the lock on one's door, the telephone in case of emergency, a flashlight when the electricity fails. The nonhuman environment also provides security symbolically. A classic example is the transitional objects of a child: a frayed blanket or a stuffed animal is a significant and important object that contributes to growth. Even adults treasure nonhuman objects that symbolize a security-giving person or situation. For example, when they establish their own home, many adults take with them from their parents' home some special object that they guard carefully for many years.

The nonhuman environment offers an opportunity for self-understanding. Love, tenderness, nurturing, or sadistic or selfish impulses can be directed toward the nonhuman environment with some degree of safety. For example, a child learns much about his capacity to nurture by caring for a puppy; an adult in moments of anger or frustration may slam down books or break a tennis racket. Such activities provide an opportunity for the individual to become consciously aware of these feelings and impulses. In addition, the individual, hopefully, comes to recognize that these emotions are good, acceptable, and a controllable part of the self. Some of the individual's assets and limitations may be tested through interaction with the nonhuman environment. Physical dexterity, problem solving, tolerance for ambiguity, and the ability to give and receive love are examples.

In addition to gaining self-understanding from the nonhuman environment, one can also gain understanding of others. Observation of another person's interaction with the nonhuman environment gives the observer considerable information about that person. Individuals tend to express feelings more freely and honestly toward the nonhuman environment than toward the human environment. Although a precise relationship cannot and should not be made, there is often some relationship. For example, an individual who is cruel to animals may not be someone we would want as a friend. The individual who asks before looking through our bookshelves may arouse a very different response.

The nonhuman environment facilitates the initial development as well as the maintenance of all performance components. Some of the examples given above emphasize the relationship between the nonhuman environment and psychological functions and social interaction. It is important to remember, however, the significance of the nonhuman environment in relationship to sensory integration, cognitive function, and neuromuscular function. In the early years a child is exposed to a vast variety of sensory stimulation from the nonhuman environment: sounds, textures, shapes, smells, to name only a few. These stimuli provide the impetus for development of sensory integrative skills. Relative to the development of cognition, the child often begins to conceptualize and learn about relationships through manipulating nonhuman objects. For example, balls are for throwing, cups are for drinking, only so many blocks will fit into a pail. Neuromotor development is enhanced through interaction with the nonhuman environment. Watching a child learn how to go up and down stairs provides ample evidence of this relationship. However, not only initial development but the continued development and maintenance of these functions is facilitated by interaction with the nonhuman environment. As noxious as it occasionally is, the nonhuman environment presents us with sensory stimuli that need to be integrated. Our continued need for cognitive stimuli is evident in the current popularity of games of strategy. We pursue such activities as jogging, swimming, and racketball to maintain neuromuscular function.

The nonhuman environment enhances the quality of life. This is particularly evident in our use of tools and various technologies. For example, most homes in the United States have running water, food is available at the local supermarket, and various means of transportation get us fairly quickly to distant locations. These conveniences allow us more time to engage in other activities that may be far more rewarding than, for example, fetching water from a well. Various tools and technologies have freed the individual to devote more time to interpersonal relationships and activities that satisfy self-actualization needs.

Similarly, in many respects, the nonhuman environment can be a source of pleasure, enjoyment, and relaxation. A walk on a quiet beach in the early evening, reading a good book, and listening to classical music are experiences many people regard as special. We treasure and enjoy many of our possessions: our home and its furnishings, a worn bathrobe we wear after a long day's work, a wall hanging we bought while visiting a foreign country. All these, too, enhance the quality of our life.

Finally, relative to human growth and development, the nonhuman environment provides relief from the human environment. At times everyone needs to be alone. In the healthy individual this need for withdrawal is periodic and temporary. While alone, the individual has an opportunity to relax, sort out feelings and ideas, plan, and recoup energy. After such a period of withdrawal the individual feels refreshed and ready for further productive interaction with the human environment.

Interaction with the nonhuman environment offers many opportunities for positive growth and development as briefly outlined above. However, the nonhuman environment may also be a source of anxiety in two different ways. One is that there appears to be a desire to be nonhuman versus a fear of regression to being nonhuman. Individuals tend to glorify that which is nonhuman. They perceive the life of plants and animals as being stable, free from anxiety and stress, without responsibility. Thus we use such expressions as "free as a bird" and "calm as a cucumber." Conversely, individuals fear return to an infantile state of nondifferentiation from the nonhuman environment. There is something innately horrible in the contemplation of not being able to think, to talk, to move. The deep response we have to the statement "She is alive but will always be a vegetable" is one indication of the fear of becoming nonhuman. Regardless of whether one knows the individual being discussed, the response is one of fear of loss of one's own humanness. Our involvement with the human environment is not always satisfying, which leads to the desire to escape and become part of the nonhuman environment. In turn this leads to a fear of regression. Thus a conflict is established, which can cause considerable anxiety.

The other source of anxiety relative to the nonhuman environment also arises out of a conflictual situation. Individuals appear to have a desire for oneness with the universe; on the other hand, individuals appear to have a desire for a sense of humanness and individuality. This is the existential conflict of wishing to be unique and different from all other objects, human or nonhuman, yet wishing to be a part of and similar to others. Relative to the latter wish, individuals seem to feel a conscious or unconscious sense of unity with the nonhuman environment. Intellectually, we know of our origin and phylogenetic development from that which is nonhuman. But even before the theory of evolution was articulated, our relationship to the nonhuman environment was expressed in myths, literature, dance, and the visual arts. To make things a bit more complex, individuals in Western society have pretty much disowned all that is perceived as "animal" in the human species. For example, euphemisms are used to speak of defecation and the natural odors of the human body. Many scientists are preoccupied with demonstrating that aside from a few biological differences, males and females of the human species are basically similar. In addition, individuals in Western society seem to be preoccupied with individuality. There is a somewhat realistic fear of being faceless in a faceless crowd, of being identified as only a number. In conclusion, the idea of the common nature of all individuals and the foundation of that nature in the nonhuman environment is sometimes threatening to the individual living in urban modern Western society.

The nonhuman environment facilitates growth and development, but it may also be the source of some natural tension. However, neither of these will occur if constructive interaction with the nonhuman environment or parts of it is impeded. Several factors may cause this to happen. First, the individual may be overly concerned with the nonhuman environment because it is excessively demanding or because it is seen as threatening or ambivalent. An example of an excessively demanding nonhuman environment is that of a young girl who must take responsibility for most of the cooking, cleaning, and laundry for a large household. This child has little opportunity to experience the nonhuman environment as a source of pleasure or an area for exploration. The nonhuman environment may seem threatening or ambivalent to an individual who subsists on the cultivation of a small plot of land. If this land is in an area where there are recurring floods and drought, the individual may view the nonhuman environment as an unfriendly and uncontrollable force.

An individual may not be comfortable in interaction with the nonhuman environment because efforts to do so are received with disfavor by significant others. For example, a child whose parents forbid him to climb trees, rollerskate, or learn to ride a bicycle for fear he might be injured comes to fear the environment. Although such a child may experience pleasure in reading or playing the piano, one major part of the nonhuman environment is not being fully utilized for growth.

Conversely, excessive need to use the nonhuman environment to gain approval from others may impede constructive use of that environment. For example, a child may perceive that his parents measure his worth by the grades he receives in school or his skill on the basketball court. Such a child is not using the nonhuman environment to facilitate well-rounded development but rather as a means to gain acceptance.

The human environment may seem so threatening to the individual that he or she uses the nonhuman environment as a means of unhealthy escape. This is different from the use of the nonhuman environment mentioned earlier. The nonhuman environment can serve as a periodic and temporary means of withdrawing from the human environment. However, this is not the situation being discussed here. The individual literally uses the nonhuman environment as a relatively permanent refuge from the human environment. For example, an individual may become preoccupied with a hobby that requires no interaction with others. Or an individual may become engrossed in the paperwork of her job to the exclusion of interacting with other people in the work setting.

Adequate use of the nonhuman environment may be impeded because the individual has come to see himself as a nonhuman object. This often takes place because the individual has been treated as if he were nonhuman by significant others. For example, this may occur when a child is raised by parents who are preoccupied with and take great pride in their collection of antique clocks. The child may well perceive that to get their attention it may be far better to be more like a clock than a human being. In many work situations, management makes the individual feel like a nonhuman object, as reflected by the expression "I feel like a cog in a wheel."

Finally, constructive interaction with the natural nonhuman environment may be impeded by technological advances that have placed a distance between the individual and nature. This is particularly true of people who live in large urban areas. Steel and concrete, the sounds of traffic, noxious odors, and air pollution are far from grass and trees, the sounds of crickets, the smell of wet earth, and clean air. When a friend tells a city dweller she is going to the country for a long weekend, there is likely to be at least a momentary feeling of envy. The need for periodic contact with nature persists in even the most confirmed urban inhabitant.

In summary, this section describes some elements of the nonhuman environment, one of the legitimate tools of occupational therapy. The discussion is concerned with three major aspects of the nonhuman environment: (a) the way in which the nonhuman environment facilitates normal growth and development, (b) the nonhuman environment as a possible source of anxiety, and (c) the ways in which constructive interaction with the nonhuman environment may be impeded.

CONSCIOUS USE OF SELF

Conscious use of self involves a planned interaction with another person in order to alleviate fear or anxiety; provide reassurance; obtain necessary information; provide information; give advice; and assist the other individual to gain more appreciation, expression, and functional use of his or her latent inner resources (14,15,47,67,134,142). Such a relationship is concerned with promoting growth and development, improving and maintaining function, and fostering a greater ability to cope with the stresses of life.

Conscious use of self may be differentiated from spontaneous response to another, the art of practice, and rapport. *Spontaneous response to another person* is typical of daily interaction with others. Such a response is often unconscious or subconscious in the sense that the individual does not preplan what specific messages will be communicated. Conversely, conscious use of self involves considerable forethought relative to the nature of a particular message and how that message is best conveyed to another individual. Conscious use of self is important in some aspects of daily life, but it is imperative in the evaluation and intervention process.

The *art of practice* as outlined in Chapter 2 is any interaction between practitioner and client which assists in diminishing the isolation of the client; reaffirms the powers of the human mind, body, and spirit; and provides the means whereby the client may discover meaning in existence. The art of practice is global or general in the sense that it is applied throughout evaluation and intervention. The conscious use of self is selective. The practitioner uses the self in different ways depending on the client's immediate needs and the various phases of the evaluation and intervention process.

Rapport is the process of establishing and maintaining a comfortable, unconstrained relationship of mutual confidence and respect between a practitioner and client. This is indeed a part of conscious use of self, but only a part. Rapport, similar to the art of practice, forms a solid substratum for evaluation and intervention. However, application of the art of practice and the establishment and maintenance of rapport *per se* are not likely to enhance a client's ability to function in the community. This is not to say that these areas are unimportant—they are very important if not crucial. But they are only the foundation for the building, not the building itself.

Conscious use of self is the manipulation of one's responses to assist a client. Depending on the situation the therapist may be supportive, permissive, accepting, cajoling, strict, demanding, or some variation on these themes. The particular response called for on a given occasion depends on the needs of the client and the frame of reference being used for the evaluation and intervention process. Conscious use of self can be compared to playing a delicate musical instrument, with the therapist as both the instrument and the musician. With skill and care the therapist uses himself to achieve the appropriate tone, pitch, harmony, tempo, rhythm, and accent. The symphony continues throughout the evaluation and intervention process. However, the message may frequently change.

The conscious use of self also involves the therapist's sensitivity to his personal response to the client. In other words, the therapist asks, How does the client make me feel? What am I experiencing? This information is valuable for it assists in assessing the client's feelings which may not be openly expressed. Through a personal response, the therapist experiences whether the client is feeling comfortable, wants to express positive feelings, is anxious, is decidedly hostile, or is acting as if the therapist is the client's nurturing grandmother. To continue the analogy of the therapist as a delicate musical instrument and musician, the therapist listens to the other musicians or ensemble to understand and know how the next note should be played.

How one develops the ability to use one's self consciously and guidelines for this process are beyond the scope of this text. Many others have described this phenomenon in great detail. Conscious use of self may take place in one-to-one interaction or in interactions with a group of clients or with those others significant to the clients. The means by which a therapist makes effective use of the self may vary from one situation to another. However, typically they include verbal dialogue, gestures, facial expressions, and "touching with care" (67; p.11).

TEACHING-LEARNING PROCESS

The teaching-learning process has been a tool of occupational therapy since its inception. Even from its informal beginnings, occupational therapy has been concerned with teaching clients how to acquire skills for living in a community with others. However, as a tool the teaching-learning process was, for some period of time, rarely mentioned in the literature and not discussed in professional circles. There are probably several reasons for this hiatus, but the major reason seems to have been concern for professional identity. Occupational therapists for a time needed to dissociate themselves from the incorrect image of being teachers of arts and crafts. However, in the process of clarifying their role, occupational therapists jettisoned the teaching-learning process, discarding more than was really necessary. To be a "therapist" was somehow better and more prestigious than helping clients to learn.

In the late 1960s occupational therapists began once again to accept the teaching-learning process as one of their major tools (33,43,59,62,63, 66,68,108,111,148). Several factors probably facilitated this process. The two major factors were (a) a marked increase in occupational therapists' self-worth and self-awareness and (b) the health professions' obsession with B. F. Skinner's theory of operant conditioning. As a result, the idea that learning was a part of any therapeutic process became respectable.

With the above brief historical survey of this somewhat mistreated tool, a few definitions may be useful. *Teaching* is the process of "instructing by precept, example or experience." According to Hilgard and Bower (62; p. 2), *learning* is a process wherein behavior "originates or is changed through reaction to an encounter situation provided that the characteristics of the change...cannot be explained on the basis of native response tendencies, maturation or temporary states of the organism (e.g., fatigue, drugs, etc.)." The term *teaching-learning process* is used here to indicate the close relationship between the teacher and the learner. An individual learns much without the aid of any formal or informal teaching. Only when the individual is unable or unlikely to learn without assistance is a teacher required. Thus the tool of teaching-learning is used only when an individual is unable to independently acquire those skills necessary for successful participation in a community with others.

Various theories of learning have been identified as part of the theoretical foundation of occupational therapy. However, teaching and learning as a tool is not based on any particular theory of learning. In its application, the tool may be based on one of the various theories of learning. For example, some frames of reference are based exclusively on operant conditioning, others are based on a psychoanalytic approach to learning, and still others use gestalt learning theory.

In addition, some frames of reference are based on postulates derived from various theories of learning. As an example both of the use of postulates from different learning theories and of what is meant by the teaching-learning process, the following outline is presented.

To facilitate the teaching-learning process a therapist:

Begins where the client is and teaches at a rate that is comfortable for the client;

Takes into consideration the client's inherent capacities, current assets and limitations, age, sex, interests, and cultural background;

Designs experiences so that the client actively participates in the learning process;

Understands the importance of reinforcement and feedback as the consequence of action;

Provides opportunity for trial and error exploration and imitation;

Allows for repetition or practice of that which is to be learned;

Acts on the knowledge that the client is more likely to attain goals that he has set rather than those set by someone else;

Encourages practice in different situations to facilitate generalization and discrimination;

Emphasizes the necessity for the client to understand what is to be learned and the reason for learning;

Plans experiences so that the client moves from simplified wholes to more complex wholes;

Encourages the client to discover inventive solutions to problems as well as more usual and typical solutions;

Is aware of individual differences as to the ways in which anxiety affects learning (111).

In summary, the teaching-learning process is one of the legitimate tools of occupational therapy. The specific teaching-learning principles or postulates used vary with the therapist's frame of reference and the learning style of a particular client.

PURPOSEFUL ACTIVITIES

Purposeful activities are doing processes directed toward a planned or hypothesized end result. In contrast, random activities are undirected and without a predetermined goal. According to Fidler (48; p. 308), an activity is purposeful only if it is congruent with "the individual's sensory, motor, cognitive, psychological and social maturation . . . developmental needs and skill readiness . . . and recognized by (the individual's) social and cultural groups as relevant to their values and needs." Purposeful activities are doing processes that involve "investigating, trying out and gaining evidence of one's capacities for experiencing, responding, managing, creating and controlling." (8).

Purposeful activity, which involves interaction with both the human and nonhuman environments, is considered to be one of the major factors that contribute to optimal growth and development (82). It has been fairly well documented that the individual has a need for mastery or competence. This need can be satisfied only through direct interaction with, apprehension of, and some influence over the human and nonhuman environment. The reader may identify with this need for mastery in recalling an experience in which one felt the "joy of being a cause, the excitement of mastery, the satisfaction of achievement" (48, p. 307).

In the maturational process purposeful activities provide an opportunity for developing sensory, neuromotor, cognitive, psychological, and social skills. Not only are these skills developed, they are also tested. Through feedback from both the human and nonhuman environments an individual learns about his or her assets, limitations, and potential. In addition, the individual also learns a good deal about the environment (35,48,65,106, 111,131,169; D. Shapiro, *unpublished observation*).

An example may be useful at this point. Remember your first lesson in learning how to drive a car. There were many known skills to be used and many new skills to be learned, all of which had to be integrated in order to respond quickly to the demands of the situation. At the beginning the car perhaps lurched forward in a halting fashion and did not stay exactly in the middle of the lane. But after a little time you began to get some idea of how the car worked, some sense of being in control. The fact that the car eventually stopped leaping about and stayed relatively in the center of the lane gave you feedback from the nonhuman environment. You also hopefully received feedback from your instructor: nonverbal feedback as her hands no longer clutched the dashboard in an act of self-preservation; verbal feedback may have come in the form of "You are doing fine." Or "All right, drive over to the side of the road." This was extremely positive feedback for it meant that your instructor really thought you could pull off to the side of the road and stop the car. In this whole process you also learned something about yourself: your ability to deal with a new situation, tolerate stress, realize this may be the last moment of your life. In addition, you learned something about your instructor; is this person supportive, vindictive, fearful, or seemingly without humor. This learning is the essence of purposeful activity.

With the above general outline of the nature and function of purposeful activities, a more specific description may be useful. Much of our understanding of the role of purposeful activities as a means to facilitate growth has come from the literature on child and adolescent development. However, with a little imagination the reader should be able to extrapolate the information provided below to growth and change throughout the life cycle.

Margaret Mead and others have emphasized that play and games are a primary factor in the socialization process. Such purposeful activities are circumscribed by the norms and values of one's particular culture of origin (131). For example, typically a culture defines acceptable roles for each sex and provides children with toys and experiences that will help them to learn these differences and develop skill in their eventual roles as an adult. The games of each culture provide an individual with an opportunity to learn acceptable ways of interacting with other members of the cultural group. In illustration, baseball was at one time considered the national pastime in the United States. Football and hockey have gained increasing popularity recently. These games differ in many ways, one of which is the degree of violence required and permitted. This perhaps says something about our society's changing norms and values relative to interpersonal relations.

Another but related factor concerning the socialization process is the importance of recognition by others of what one has learned or accomplished through engaging in purposeful activity (48). A child who figures out how to form an arch out of flat, interlocking blocks is much more likely to continue to explore other forms of construction if the child's first discovery and execution are greeted with excitement and applause. The pleasure of learning something new, the delight in mastery, is often a hollow and short-lived victory if it is not shared with and recognized by others who are significant to the individual. What was learned, discovered, or gained for the moment is often lost for it is not considered important by the members of one's cultural group.

There are two interrelated ways of viewing purposeful activities as the bases for socialization and skill development in childhood and adolescence. Moore and Anderson (106) focus primarily on play, games, and involvement in arts and crafts as significant in the developmental process. However, they do not describe any particular sequence. Mary Reilly (131), on the other hand, describes how socialization takes place through the sequence of play, arts and crafts, games, and chores.

Moore and Anderson describe the process of solving various types of puzzles as providing an opportunity for individuals to see themselves as causal agents. Solving a puzzle engenders a sense of being in control of the situation at hand. Conversely, games of chance help individuals to understand that there are events over which they have no control, thus appreciating the unknowable or uncontrollable elements that influence some aspects of life experience. Games of strategy require individuals to attend to the motivation, thinking, feelings, and behavior of others. The ability to focus on these aspects of another person prepares us to deal with negotiating in real life situations. Involvement in various arts and crafts is seen as helping individuals not only to appreciate and understand aesthetics but, more importantly, to make normative judgments. Through arts and crafts, individuals have an opportunity to evaluate what they and others are able to do or produce. This is a beginning step in the formation of a value system, a system that is personal but also founded in one's cultural group.

Reilly views individual play as an opportunity to explore the self and the environment with minimal outside constraints. In this type of play there are no rules or imposed structures; it is an adventure in examining, investigating, questioning, and searching. Arts and crafts, the next step in the sequence of socialization, are seen as providing a structure for self-evaluation imposed by the nonhuman environment. Individuals are able to determine their competence by reference to the end product produced. This type of evaluation is different from that mentioned by Moore and Anderson. They suggest that arts and crafts provide an opportunity to learn something about making normative judgments. Reilly, on the other hand, considers arts and crafts as a means for evaluating one's competence relative to understanding of and having some control over the nonhuman environment. A simple example of the latter is learning how much glue is needed to secure one object to another or figuring out how to refinish a chair bought at a garage sale. Reilly considers that playing games with others provides an opportunity to learn the idea of rules. Through involvement in games the individual learns that there are principles which govern acceptable behavior in a particular social system. Through participation in games the individual learns how to relate to, share, and cooperate with peers. In addition, within the context of the rules of various games, the individual also learns something about dealing with an adversary, competition, and how to win. Finally, Reilly describes chores or tasks imposed by another person as the basis for learning how to relate to those in authority. Chores also help an individual to understand that there are unpleasant tasks which must be learned and performed on a regular basis. For example, a child may be required to cut the grass and take out the garbage. Neither of these chores is pleasant. But such tasks teach the child something about authority and that only a part of life is play.

Routine purposeful activities are so much a part of our daily life and so ordinary in nature that they often go unnoticed (35). One thinks little about getting out of bed in the morning, making the coffee, and taking a quick shower. We think so little of these activities that it often seems that we are performing them almost in our sleep, which at times may be the case.

Purposeful activities tend to be given attention primarily in the negative, when something goes amiss in the usual or expected process (D. Shapiro, *unpublished observation*). An individual may cease to perform typical purposeful activities. For example, a friend, usually somewhat meticulous, may repeatedly arrive late to work dressed in a disheveled manner. One's first response other than general concern would be to question the individual's physical and/or emotional well-being. Everyday purposeful activities are also given attention when they can be performed only with considerable thought and effort. For example, if one's dominant hand and arm are immobilized in a cast, such tasks as dressing and putting in contact lenses become difficult and time consuming. Finally, we tend to note activities that appear to be purposeful for the individual performing the activity but the purpose cannot be deduced by the observer. One may, for example, observe an individual taking all of his pictures and prints off the wall and depositing them in large garbage bags. There may be a logical reason for this, such as that the individual's apartment is going to be painted. On the other hand, the individual may be engaged in this activity because the pictures and prints are to be thrown away for they remind him of a close relationship that has just been terminated. In either case the observer needs to question the individual to discover the purpose of the activity.

Purposeful activities "permeate the fabric of daily living" (35; p. 9). They are such a part of our life that their significance and importance often go unnoticed. Yet without purposeful activities there would be little to differentiate the human experience from that of nonhuman objects. Indeed, one could say that without purposeful activity there would be no human experience.

Purposeful activities may be realistic, symbolic, or a combination of the two. In the example given above, the individual who was taking pictures and prints down from the wall so that his apartment could be painted was engaging in an activity considered realistic. The individual throwing away his pictures and prints was engaging in a symbolic activity. Careful preparation of a meal for a special person is an example of a realistic and symbolic activity: it is realistic in the sense of shopping, cooking, and setting an attractive table; it is symbolic in the sense of expressing love and wanting to nurture the other individual.

A short digression on the topic of symbolism might clarify the nature of symbolic activities (22,26,47,73,74,85,101,108,143). A *symbol* is an action, object, image, or word that has special complexities of meanings in addition to its conventional or obvious meaning. Although it can be explained in some detail after study, a symbol always has unknown or hidden elements. For example, a person might be able to give a fairly good explanation of her pleasure in polishing the silver tea service that originally belonged to her great-grandmother. However, something about the process and the feelings it engenders cannot be described.

In this way a symbol is different from a sign. A *sign* is an action, object, image, or word that stands for another action, object, image, or word. There is no mystery to a sign; it can be easily understood. Symbols have an emotional component, whereas affect is rarely associated with signs. Some examples of signs are nodding one's head to indicate agreement, a poster in the bookstore announcing the availability of a current best seller, and a map indicating the routes of the various subway trains in Boston.

Symbols may be universal, cultural, or idiosyncratic. Actually, most symbols have all three elements. A symbol is universal to the extent that either the form or content of the symbol has been shared by a variety of cultural groups widely different in time and place. For example, the form of a circle has been used to symbolize peace or unity by many cultural groups. The idea of evil and the life cycle are common themes in many cultural groups. These themes may be symbolized in many different ways, in myths, visual arts, and ceremonies, for example.

A symbol is considered to be cultural when it is shared and understood by most members of a cultural group. Cultural symbols may endure for a long time or be transient in nature. For example, the flag of the United

States has served as a cultural symbol for all citizens of this country—regardless of political orientation— for a considerable period of time. On the other hand, men wearing their hair long, a cultural symbol of the early 1970s, has lost the significance which it had at that time.

Finally, idiosyncratic symbols are those symbols which are unique to an individual or to a small group of individuals. For example, an individual may collect owl figurines or prefer the color blue. A family may consider the last Thursday of November to be Thanksgiving Day only if a casserole of squash, peanuts, and sour cream is served.

In considering any potentially symbolic activity (and most activities do have such a potential), it is instructive to look at the three components outlined above. Through exploring the universal, cultural, and idiosyncratic symbolic meaning of an activity we are often better able to understand the activity and the individual engaging in that activity. In conclusion, then, purposeful activities have a realistic quality, but they often also have a symbolic quality.

Purposeful activities have been a part of occupational therapy since its inception (see references on p. 1). Initially they were used in two different ways: (a) as a means of providing temporary relief from physical pain, anxiety, depression, and boredom; and (b) to help individuals to develop, relearn, or maintain an apparently natural rhythm between work, play, and rest. While using and studying purposeful activities, occupational therapists learned far more about their potential for restoring and maintaining function. Through participation in a wide variety of purposeful activities the individual accumulates "a store of action experiences essential for human function; a reservoir of experiences gathered from direct engagement with the environment" (48; p. 306). The use of purposeful activities as a tool for intervention has become increasingly important as greater emphasis has been placed on verbal skills or language in our culture. There is a tendency to deal in the abstract rather than the concrete (35). It is fine, for example, to know the general principle for hanging wall shelves or reassembling a kitchen step stool. However, in executing these activities one truly understands the principles and one's capacity to apply abstract knowledge to actual situations. When thought does not lead to some type of action, critical opportunities for learning are lost (48). In addition, the individual does not gain sufficient experience in understanding the consequence of action.

There are many individuals who, because of past experience or the lack of experience, are fearful of engaging in purposeful activity. Such individuals often have considerable verbal skill. They are comfortable talking about something, but when there is a distinct demand to engage in a purposeful activity related to their knowledge base they become fearful. Such individuals are apprehensive that they might demonstrate incompetence. They have had little experience with the task at hand and little experience with the consequences of success or failure relative to purposeful activities. In the extreme, individuals who lack experience in engaging in purposeful activities tend to view themselves as inept or inadequate in many areas of human function (48).

As used in occupational therapy, purposeful activities may be simulated or natural (82). Simulated activities are engaged in within a clinical setting and are designed to develop skills that can be used in the community (35). This is not meant to imply that there is anything artificial or unreal about simulated purposeful activities. They are organized, goal directed, and based on a particular theoretical system. An analogy of this type of purposeful activity is the various simulated activities designed to prepare the astronauts for their ventures into space. To prepare an individual for participation in the community, a simulated activity must (a) be relevant to the development of skills the individual will need for successful participation in the community; (b) arouse and sustain the individual's interest in the learning process; and (c) resemble as closely as possible the activity patterns the individual is likely to encounter in the community (35). An example of the latter is helping a person learn how to independently dress and engage in other areas of personal hygiene shortly after waking in the morning rather than attempting to teach these activities sometime in the middle of the afternoon.

A natural purposeful activity is one that takes place in the community. This type of activity may occur in the company of the therapist, with fellow clients, or the client may engage in the activity independently. Some examples of natural purposeful activities are going roller skating in a local park, applying for a job, and helping one's children with their homework. Natural activities in which the therapist is not involved are sometimes referred to as prescribed activities (48; J. Pierce, *personal communication*). Such activities are agreed on by the client and therapist for the purpose of testing and practicing new skills. In such a situation the therapist serves as a resource person providing support and guidance relative to problem solution and reinforcement. Typically the intervention process begins with simulated purposeful activities and moves in the direction of natural purposeful activities. This, however, may not always be the case. Natural purposeful activities may be used initially and throughout the intervention process. Examples of the latter are assisting a somewhat anxious and mildly depressed new mother with infant care, and altering the dynamics of the family constellation through guiding the client's direct involvement in the situation to be mastered.

In summary, purposeful activity, one of the tools of occupational therapy, provides individuals with an opportunity to develop various skills necessary for participation in the community and to learn about their strengths and limitations. Purposeful activities are goal oriented and emphasize the idea of learning through doing.

ACTIVITY GROUPS

Activity groups are primary groups made up of and designed to assist individuals who share common concerns or problems related to the acquisition or maintenance of performance components or occupational performance. Activities are either an integral part of the groups' here-and-now interaction or a specific gestalt of activities, engaged in by group members outside of the context of the groups. In the latter case the gestalt of activities becomes the focus for group discussion. A *primary group* is a face-to-face organization of people who cooperate for certain common ends, who have confidence in and some degree of affection for each other, and who are aware of their similarities and bonds of association (111).

The concept and use of activity groups evolved from an integration of three different theoretical systems. The first is the role of purposeful activities in the development and maintenance of skills needed for successful participation in the community. The second element comes from study of the dynamics of small groups (27,60,104,119). The third element is derived from identification of those factors in small groups that can be manipulated to bring about positive change in group members (39,89,96,140,163,167). The latter, sometimes referred to as the general therapeutic factors of small groups, are used in verbal therapy groups as well as activity groups. The dynamics of small groups and general therapeutic factors of small groups are not discussed in this text. Each is a large area of study in and of itself and is covered in other texts.

Properly designed activity groups have several components that contribute to evaluation and intervention (19,23,32,44,55,57,61,76,79,86,90,97,98, 102,111,122,164). Activity groups provide a "laboratory for living: a microcosm of life, learning and work." *Laboratory* is used here to denote a situation in which something may be seen, studied, and understood as it occurs rather than in retrospect. Learning tends to occur through experience in contrast to information gained through a more didactic approach. A useful analogy is the first time one sees a frog's heart beating in a biology lab. Although one read about the phenomenon in a textbook, it may have been just one more fact to be memorized. But the image of the frog's beating heart is not easily forgotten. A laboratory experience, then, can be a powerful source for learning.

Activity groups provide a setting similar to that found in the normal developmental process. Much learning takes place through involvement in a variety of purposeful activities in various primary groups, including family, friends, school, and work. Learning occurs naturally in the process of shared activities rather than through verbal discussion only. We acquired some rudiments of table manners at the family dining room table; we gained some knowledge of how to budget our time when we had our first summer job.

Activity groups provide a degree of structure and organization which is useful to many clients. Because activity groups involve a doing process as well as discussion, an individual is given an opportunity to integrate and use presently available skills. Thus an individual who is fearful of engaging in activities has an opportunity to participate in the group on a verbal level. Conversely, individuals who are shy or who lack verbal skills may become part of the group primarily through participation in the activity. This element of activity groups facilitates initial comfort and involvement. With such involvement the individual is then able to begin to acquire skills in various areas of dysfunction.

Another way in which activity groups provide structure and organization is that their framework allows expression of ideas and feelings within known limits. The activity is sufficiently concrete so as to focus group members' thoughts on the problems and issues which are the specific goals of that activity group. For example, if the goal of the group is to develop work habits, group members know they are participating in the group to practice certain skills only. They are not there to acquire leisure skills nor are they there to share problems related to family interaction.

Activity groups provide an opportunity for constructive use of the nonhuman environment. It is often easier for the individual to focus on the activity rather than on interpersonal relationships. In turn, the activity may provide a means of identification with the group because the group shares a common set of tasks. The reaction of others in such interactions as response to a request for assistance may be assessed first in relationship to the activity. This gives the individual some idea of how other group members may respond when assistance is sought relative to intrapersonal or interpersonal problems. Individuals who have difficulty mastering or manipulating the nonhuman environment are able to problem solve together within the context of an activity. In illustration, a group of quadriplegic clients may gain skill in using power-driven wheelchairs through involvement in various contests and games that require maneuvering their wheelchairs. Later this same group of clients may feel sufficiently comfortable with each other to share their fears about being disabled. The shared need to master a nonhuman object often assists clients to develop a sense of commonality with others.

Activity groups provide an opportunity to focus on the doing process. As previously mentioned, some individuals have problems relative to doing. They are often able to talk about engaging in a variety of purposeful activities but are unable to follow through on the performance level. Activity groups facilitate collaboration in identifying difficulties in doing. The specific request to participate in an activity minimizes denial or rationalization relative to actual proficiency in performance. Attempts to evade responsibility for contributing to task completion, for example, are easily demonstrated when group members are mutually dependent on each other for task completion.

Finally, activity groups provide a tangible means of measuring the progress of each group member and the progress of the group as a whole. The activity is a concrete reality factor against which the individual can measure achievement and growth. For the individual, positive change can be demonstrated by the degree to which the individual was able to contribute to completing the activity over a period of time. For the group as a whole, positive change may be measured by the degree of movement toward completing a particular activity or the increasing complexity of the activities which the group selects and completes.

The above discussion of activity groups has been general in nature and refers to all activity groups. However, there are many types of activity groups. For example, there is considerable difference in a group designed to increase the sensory integrative skills of 6-year-old children and a group designed to explore intrapsychic processes. There is no commonly accepted system for categorizing activity groups in the literature, so they tend to be labeled by a particular goal, such as "work adjustment group" or by the activity used, such as "cooking group." This leads to some confusion as to the nature of the group. Thus a tentative taxonomy of activity groups is offered below. This classification is based on some similarity in the group goals, the types of frames of reference that may be used as the basis for a particular group, clients who may benefit from participation, the role of the therapist, and activities used. Out of necessity this discussion is brief. There are six major categories of activity groups, although some of these categories are further subdivided.

Evaluation groups are designed to assess an individual's ability to function within a group in terms of both interpersonal skills and relationship to a shared activity. Such a group provides information for both client and therapist about the client's capacities and limitations relative to participation in a group situation. This type of group is only concerned with evaluation, and thus no planned intervention takes place. The specifics of the areas of function and dysfunction to be evaluated depend on the frame of reference being utilized. The therapist is primarily an observer and becomes an active participant only if a potentially dangerous or destructive situation arises. The activity, selected by the therapist, is any short-term activity that requires group planning and collaborative interaction for completion.

Task-oriented groups are designed to increase the individual's awareness of how intrapsychic phenomena (perception of self and others) influence interaction with others and the process of doing. Further, they are designed to teach members more functional ways of interaction based on this new awareness. To be suited for this type of group, clients must have at least a fair amount of verbal skill. The major role of the therapist is to assist group members in exploring the relationship between thoughts, feelings, and actions and to suggest ways in which an individual may identify, practice, and learn new patterns of behavior. Suitable activities are those directed toward creating an end product or a demonstrable service for the group as a whole or for persons outside of the group (44).

Developmental groups are designed to teach group interaction skills only. They are based on frames of reference that describe the learning of group interaction skill as being developmentally stage specific. Thus various sub-categories of groups are included in this category. For example, an individual may be placed in an elementary developmental group if he or she has minimal skill in relating to others in a group. A more advanced level of developmental group would be used to assist a client who had acquired some ability to engage in a variety of groups as a mature, contributing member. The role of the therapist varies with the level of the subgroup. However, the therapist's role in meeting individual needs and in selecting suitable activities tends to diminish as one moves from the lowest to the highest level of developmental groups. Suitable activities tend to become more long-term, collaborative, and complex as one moves toward the advanced developmental groups (111).

Thematic groups are designed to assist clients in gaining knowledge, skills, and/or attitudes necessary for performing a circumscribed set of activities. These may include performance components such as sensory integration or neuromuscular function or occupational performances such as activities of daily living or recreational/leisure skills. Further, the goal of thematic groups is to assist individuals to carry out these activities independently within the protective environment of the clinical center or residence. The role of the therapist varies depending on the needs and level of sophistication of the group. On one end of the continuum, the therapist may be highly supportive, directive, and didactic. On the other end of the continuum, the therapist may serve primarily as a resource person and knowledgeable guide. Depending on the knowledge, skills, and attitudes to be taught, suitable activities would be described as simulated as that term was used in the section on purposeful activities.

Topical groups are designed to reach the same goals as outlined for thematic groups. The major difference is that they are designed to assist group members to carry out these activities independently within the community. There are two types of topical groups. The first is an *anticipatory group*, which is focused on discussion regarding a gestalt of related activities that group members expect to engage in in the near future. These activities may be relatively new to the client, or the client may need or plan to engage in these activities in a different manner. An example of an anticipatory group is a pre-discharge group in which members discuss people's reactions to their physical disability or how to seek help in entering a building not readily accessible to a physically disabled individual. The other type of topical group, a *concurrent group*, is focused on a gestalt of related activities which the client is actually carrying out in the community. An example of a concurrent group is a parent group, whose members are actively engaged in child rearing. The therapist's role in an anticipatory group is to help group members to identify various aspects of the activity which need to be considered prior to engaging in the activity. Possible problem areas are discussed followed by identifying a number of feasible solutions. In a concurrent group the therapist helps group members to share experiences with each other and to give each other feedback and suggestions. The therapist often also prescribes useful activities.

Instrumental groups are designed to meet health needs and/or to maintain function. No major positive change is anticipated or expected. Individuals who cannot independently meet health needs or who need encouragement in the maintainance of function are good candidates for an instrumental group. The role of the therapist is to design activity experiences that will meet the individuals' needs relative to the goals described above. Suitable activities are essentially selected on the basis of the health needs that require satisfaction and the areas of function to be maintained.

The six categories of activity groups described above should be viewed as somewhat arbitrary and not as discrete entities. For example, a particular group may have elements of a thematic group and a topical group. The categories are described to facilitate an understanding of the various types of activity groups and to aid in communication.

Finally, the essence of activity groups can be further clarified by comparing these groups to verbal groups. (See references for general therapeutic factors in small groups and references for activity groups.) There is no sharp, definitive contrast between activity groups and verbal groups. Rather, there are degrees of variation along three different continuums: centrality of activity, immediacy of events, and circumscribed focus. *Centrality of activities* refers to the degree to which group members are involved in a shared purposeful activity. Activity groups tend to cluster at the high or positive end of this continuum. Activity groups are concerned with a doing, action-oriented process as opposed to talking about such a process in a relatively abstract manner. Manipulation of and interaction with the non-human environment is an important component of activity groups. In contrast, verbal groups tend to be concerned with discussion about intrapersonal and interpersonal interactions. The individual's involvement in everyday activities is usually of far less concern. Interaction with the nonhuman environment tends to be minor.

Immediacy of events refers to the degree to which a group focuses on here-and-now events or events likely to occur in the immediate future as opposed to past events. Activity groups tend to focus on current and near future events. Verbal groups tend to give far more attention to past events.

The third continuum, the degree of *circumscribed* focus, refers to the specificity of group goals and legitimate areas of discussion. Activity groups tend to have fairly well-defined goals and legitimate areas of discussion. For example, an activity group may be primarily concerned with how to use and budget one's time or how to find suitable housing. Verbal groups tend to have more general goals and legitimate areas of discussion. For example, the goal of a verbal group may be to increase self-awareness; in such a group few if any areas of human experience would be considered unsuitable for discussion.

Activity groups and verbal groups may vary along other dimensions, but the three dimensions described above perhaps give some flavor of the differences between these two types of therapeutic groups. However, it is important to remember that these are variations on three different continuums. No one arbitrary factor distinguishes activity groups from verbal groups.

In summary, activity groups use purposeful activities to assess an individual's assets and limitations relative to the ability to be a productive member of a variety of groups. In addition, activity groups use purposeful activities to facilitate the development and maintenance of performance components and occupational performance.

ACTIVITY ANALYSIS AND SYNTHESIS

Purposeful activities and activity groups cannot be designed to meet evaluation and intervention needs without analysis and synthesis of activities.

Activity analysis is the process of examining an activity to distinguish its component parts. *Activity synthesis* is the process of combining component parts of the human and nonhuman environment so as to design an activity suitable for evaluation or intervention relative to performance components and occupational performance (35,47,65,123,150).

The occupational therapy model gives legitimacy to activity analysis and synthesis as a tool used by occupational therapists. The model, however, specifies only the definition and need for activity analysis and synthesis, not specific conceptual frameworks for analysis and synthesis. Conceptual frameworks are provided within the literature of occupational therapy, primarily in published frames of reference.

The need for a conceptual framework for activity analysis and synthesis may require further clarification. Analysis or synthesis of any aspect of the human or nonhuman environment can take place only within a system of classification that is at least tentative. For example, one cannot analyze a bicycle without having some idea of what aspect of the bicycle is to be assessed or the purpose of that assessment. One could analyze a bicycle, for instance, relative to its being a mode of transportation, how to teach someone to ride it, or in terms of aesthetic design. Without a conceptual framework, analysis tends to be primarily speculation. Similarly, without a conceptual framework, the process of synthesis lacks direction. For example, one may be asked to make a cake. If the individual has only a vague idea of what a cake is and is unaware of the properties of the ingredients normally used in cake making, it is highly unlikely that what comes out of the oven will be a cake.

Each profession often has its own conceptual framework for looking at the varied aspects of different phenomena. For example, a graphic artist and an educator will analyze a new textbook differently. To guide his analysis a graphic artist may use such concepts as quality of illustration, size of type and page composition. An educator is more likely to use such concepts as content accuracy, organization of material, and level of abstraction necessary for comprehension. Similarly, there are various ways of synthesizing information about the human and nonhuman environment. For example, an engineer synthesizes metal for a steel girder and the shell of an airplane in very different ways. The engineer's synthesis must take into consideration among other factors, the various types of stresses to which each of the metals will be subjected.

Analysis and synthesis in occupational therapy are concerned with the study and fabrication of purposeful activities. Both study and fabrication take into consideration the human and nonhuman components of the activity. The purpose of activity analysis and synthesis, as mentioned previously, is to determine what activities are most appropriate for evaluation and intervention. There appear to be two different approaches to activity analysis and synthesis in occupational therapy. For the purpose of this discussion, these are referred to as generic and restricted.

Generic activity analysis and synthesis is based on a conceptual framework drawn from the domain of concern of the profession. The full spectrum of all aspects of the domain of concern—performance components, age, occupational performance, environment—is taken into consideration. Thus, for example, an activity is assessed relative to the neuromotor requirements necessary to perform the activity (e.g., muscles involved, direction of resistance, degree of coordination). An activity is assessed relative to its vocational application or potential for use in recreation, as well as its acceptability by various cultural groups. The Activity Analysis Form in Hopkins and Smith (65) and the Activity Analysis Outline in Cynkin (35) are two recent illustrations of a generic conceptual framework for activity analysis and synthesis.

Generic conceptual frameworks have two major deficits as a guide for activity analysis and synthesis. One is that they tend to be oriented primarily to the intervention process to the exclusion of the evaluation process. Few guidelines are provided for assessing whether an activity will elicit those behaviors which indicate if an individual is in a state of function or dysfunction in the various performance components or occupational performances.

However, more significantly, generic conceptual frameworks tend to provide no guidelines for activity synthesis. It is necessary, of course, to analyze; but what does one do with this information? Activity analysis helps one to understand the elements of a particular activity or many different activities. However, without direction relative to synthesis, the process is arrested in mid-course. Activity analysis, then, comes to be an exercise with no discernible purpose; it becomes a random activity.

Restricted activity analysis and synthesis is based on a conceptual framework drawn from a particular frame of reference (65). There are as many different systems of classification, then, for activity analysis and synthesis as there are frames of reference. This is in contrast to the generic orientation, which offers only one system of classification. An example of the conceptual framework provided by different frames of reference for activity analysis and synthesis may be useful. In looking at the intervention possibilities of taking a walk in the scarlet and amber woods of autumn, the therapist using an analytic frame of reference would look at the stimuli available for association to color and seasonal change, whereas the therapist using a rehabilitative frame of reference would assess the roughness of the terrain and the number of low hanging branches.

In the use of restricted conceptual frameworks, activity analysis and synthesis is separated into a particular activity's potential for evaluation and its potential for intervention. The behaviors indicative of function and dysfunction of a particular frame of reference form the bases for activity analysis and synthesis relative to evaluation. The postulates regarding intervention of a particular frame of reference form the bases for activity analysis and synthesis relative to intervention (108).

Before they can be evaluated, most phenomena must be measurable. In other words, as discussed in Chapter 2, the phenomena must be defined in operational terms. Phenomena may be measured by criteria which indicate the presence or absence of the phenomena. Or, more typically, phenomena may be measured by criteria which indicate the degree to which the phenomena are present. In the latter case the phenomena can then be said to exist on a continuum. Obvious examples are temperature and age.

The word *continuum* as used in the phrase "function-dysfunction continuums" connotes the same meaning as in the above paragraph. Simply stated if a person is assessed as being at one end of a particular continuum, the individual is considered to be functional in that particular area of human activity. The opposite is true if the person is assessed as being at the other end of the continuum. The operational definition of a particular function-dysfunction continuum is the "behaviors indicative of function and dysfunction" outlined for that continuum.

Evaluation of most areas of human function involves a sampling of behavior from which one may, at some risk, make a statement about the individual's capacity in that particular area (75). Classroom tests are an example of the sampling of behavior aspect of evaluation. Another important aspect of evaluation is that the process must provide an opportunity for the individual to exhibit these specific types of behaviors. Obviously, the evaluator must know what these behaviors are in order to design an adequate evaluation (75).

Based on these statements regarding evaluation, activities are analyzed relative to their probability of eliciting behaviors indicative of function and dysfunction as enumerated in a particular frame of reference. Activities are synthesized based on knowledge of the gestalt of behaviors the therapist wishes to observe. An illustration of synthesis is selecting an activity for evaluation that is likely to elicit a number of different behaviors indicative of function and dysfunction rather than an activity that is likely to elicit only one such behavior.

Postulates regarding intervention of a particular frame of reference form the basis for activity analysis and synthesis relative to intervention. Postulates regarding intervention, ideally, state the nature, quantity, quality, and sequence of interaction with the human and nonhuman environment, which is considered to be instrumental in bringing about positive change or maintaining some area of human function. Thus activities are analyzed according to whether and to what degree they embody components of the stated characteristics. For example, a postulate may state that range of joint motion is enhanced by slowly increasing the degree to which the joint is required to move beyond its current range. Activities would then be analyzed with respect to the degree which they could be graded relative to the range of motion required for a particular joint.

Activities for intervention are synthesized to be as consistent as possible with the entire postulate regarding intervention for a specific area of dysfunction. For example, a postulate might state that form perception is enhanced through visual, tactile, and proprioceptive exploration of objects. After analysis the therapist would design an activity or a series of activities that provided the greatest opportunity for visual, tactile, and proprioceptive exploration of a variety of objects.

Restrictive conceptual frameworks for activity analysis and synthesis are derived from specific frames of reference. As such, they are only as complete as the frame of reference on which they are based. If a frame of reference provides only vague behaviors indicative of function and dysfunction, then the conceptual framework for activity analysis and synthesis relative to activities suitable for evaluation will be vague. The same is true if the postulates regarding intervention of a frame of reference are inadequate: the conceptual framework for analysis and synthesis of activities for intervention will be inadequate.

Regardless of whether the practitioner is more comfortable with a generic or a restricted approach to activity analysis and synthesis, there are two precautionary notes. To analyze or synthesize an activity with knowledge and skill, one must know the activity. One should know the materials, tools, and processes involved. Ideally, the therapist has actually engaged in the activity to be analyzed and synthesized or at least studied the activity in great detail (35).

The other precautionary note is to be specific about the nature of the activity to be analyzed and synthesized. One can neither study nor design an activity in the abstract. For example, it is almost impossible to analyze "working with clay." Analysis could continue far into the therapist's well-earned years of retirement. It is far better to analyze "working with clay using the slab method" or "making a pinch pot." Similarly, in synthesis of an activity one cannot simply decide that weaving would be an excellent activity. More specificity is needed. Weaving what? A basket, rug, or fine wool scarf? And what is the interpersonal environment in which this weaving will take place? Specificity of the activity greatly enhances the process of analysis and synthesis.

CONCLUSION

In summary, this chapter describes the legitimate tools of occupational therapy—the nonhuman environment, conscious use of self, the teaching-learning process, purposeful activities, activity groups, and activity analysis and synthesis. With completion of this chapter a model for occupational therapy has been outlined. However, before this section is closed, a final chapter is included to compare the model presented here with other efforts to give unity to the diverse elements of occupational therapy.

11 / Other Integrative Ideas for Occupational Therapy

In the past several years the profession of occupational therapy has sought to identify those elements which will provide a sense of wholeness and unity to the profession. There are several reasons for this preoccupation at this particular time. One reason appears to be the increasing specialization in occupational therapy. This process has been taking place almost since the formal beginning of the profession. However, specialization has accelerated rapidly in the last 10 years and has recently been recognized in the formation of specialty groups within the formal structure of the American Occupational Therapy Association. With the increase in specialization there is the question of what is common to all areas which makes them a part of occupational therapy (4,82).

The second reason is related to the current social environment in which occupational therapy exists. With the present high degree of social change many professions, including occupational therapy, seek some sense of stability for the present and direction for the future. To counteract the uncertainty of accelerated social change there is often a search for one's "roots." This phenomenon arises out of the belief that knowledge of historical origin will provide guidance for the present and future (145).

Finally, concern for the unity of occupational therapy arises from the self-doubt that is endemic to professions. Self-doubt is not peculiar to occupational therapy. Occupational therapy probably takes the process a bit more seriously than other professions because of its youthful inexperience in dealing with this natural part of growth and development. The self-questioning of a profession occurs in cycles and provides a healthy means for reexamination, revitalization, and change.

Thus there are legitimate reasons for occupational therapy's search for unity and wholeness. It is, within limits, a productive preoccupation. In this search occupational therapists have used such terms as *theoretical framework, unifying concepts, theory, paradigm, basic beliefs, hypothesis, theoretical base, frame of reference, model,* and *philosophical assumptions.* However, these terms are rarely defined and often used as if one term had the same meaning as another term. If the above listed terms are defined they are defined only within the context of a particular published paper. No attention is given to the fact the term was defined in a far different manner in previously published occupational therapy literature. This lack of definitions or use of conflicting definitions tends to confuse the reader. The discussion of other integrative ideas to be presented shortly is thus based on the authors' interpretation of the literature.

Another problem in reading the literature is that there seem to be two apparently different orientations to the development of integrative ideas: identification of unifying elements and identification of the uniqueness of occupational therapy. However, on closer reading it is difficult to discern the difference between these orientations. Thus these orientations are treated as similar in the following discussion.

Finally, only those integrative ideas addressed to the profession as a whole are discussed. Although integrative ideas addressed to one area of specialization are of considerable importance to the profession, they were not developed to provide unity for the entire profession.

COMMON THEMES

The term *common themes* is used to differentiate this section from the following section. Common themes are integrative ideas that have been proposed in the literature as a means of providing unity to the profession. Several authors have written about one or more of these themes either in the same book or article or over a period of time in different books or articles. Thus it is important to remember that these themes have been intertwined in the literature in various combinations. In addition, no attempt has been made to present these themes in any historical sequence. They are so intertwined that finding the beginning of each thread is a task best left to skilled historians.

With this introduction, six common themes are briefly discussed:

Alternatives to the medical model were originally proposed when it became readily apparent that occupational therapists were not concerned with diagnosis of disease or eliminating pathology. Thus the content of the medical model did not, in any realistic way, relate to the occupational therapy process (129). One alternative proposed is the *health model*, which emphasizes occupational therapists' concern for using a client's assets (72, 82,132). Rather than focus on limitations or dysfunction, the occupational therapist is concerned with function. Emphasis is placed on working with populations not typically found in a clinical setting, prevention, and maximum use of community resources in the evaluation and intervention process.

Another alternative to the medical model is the *biopsychosocial model*. This is an initial attempt to articulate the structure of a model and the content of such a model for occupational therapy. Its only possible redeeming value is that it provided part of the ancestry for the occupational therapy model outlined in this text (112).

Identification of *philosophical assumptions* is another common theme. Efforts directed to this area have primarily focused on the philosophical assumptions of those active in the promotion of occupational therapy at the time of its formal beginning. Adolph Meyers and Eleanor Clark Slagle are often used as primary sources. Concern for identifying philosophical assumptions appears to have two different motives. One is the need to seek out the roots of the profession. The other is for clarification: once the profession's philosophical assumptions are specifically stated, other aspects of the profession can be more easily identified and defined (38,70,103, 145,146,169).

The need for a *theoretical foundation* for the profession is a constantly recurring subject in the literature. At times concern for identifying a theoretical foundation that is unique in its parts as well as its totality is paramount. At other times concern is expressed about the lack of organization and boundaries. Still at other times there is simply a call for additional and more definitive research. The diversity of the theoretical foundation of occupational therapy is not always recognized.

Occupational performance is another common theme. There is a focus on activities of daily living, work (including play), recreation/leisure, and temporal adaptation as being the essence of the occupational therapy process. These areas are seen as the core of the profession's domain of concern rather than as forming one part of the parameters of the domain of concern. The proponents of this theme tend to focus on various social roles and the need to develop skills relative to the individual's required social roles (25,29, 41,77,78,127,129,130).

Human growth and development is seen by many authors as a key to uniting the various areas of specialization of occupational therapy. As used in the literature, human growth and development can be equated with age (chronological and developmental), which forms one part of the parameter of the domain of concern as presented in this text. Those who identify human growth and development as of primary significance consider this factor to form the core of the profession's domain of concern. Considerable attention is given to infancy, childhood, and adolescence in the literature. However, the theme, in its broadest perspective, takes all age groups into consideration (80,91,92,128,131).

Finally, *purposeful activity* has been frequently mentioned in the literature as a unifying factor for the profession. This is not surprising in that purposeful activity is a hallmark that serves as a point of identity for the practitioners of occupational therapy. However, when purposeful activity is discussed as a unifying factor, the domain of concern of the profession tends to be only vaguely stated (35,48,56,123,128; D. Shapiro, *unpublished observation*).

These six common themes are without question important to the understanding of occupational therapy. Thus they are all included in the occupational therapy model. Proponents of the various themes may not necessarily agree as to how and where these various ideas are placed in the model, but every effort has been made to give these themes the attention and prominence they deserve.

In a more negative vein, each theme taken individually is unidimensional and thus does not reflect the variety and richness of the profession. Some of these themes have been combined in the literature, but the end result often confuses rather than clarifies, particularly for the student or novice therapist. The occupational therapy model as presented provides no new or additional information about the occupational therapy process. Indeed, the content of the model is drawn, for the most part, directly from the occupational therapy literature. The model simply provides a structure for the major common themes, outlined above, and for many of the minor themes.

PARADIGM

The concept of paradigm has been suggested by Mary Reilly and others as an integrative idea for occupational therapy (129,130). Paradigm is treated separately in this chapter because it is on a different conceptual level than the common themes outlined in the previous section. Common themes are, as the name implies, threads of ideas that are paramount in the literature of occupational therapy. In contrast, the concept of paradigm refers to a structure or a way of organizing data.

The concept of paradigm comes from the work of Kuhn (87), who defines paradigm in a number of ways. The following definition is, therefore, a synthesis. A paradigm is the typical way in which an academic discipline defines its current theoretical system, field of study, methods of research, and standards for acceptable solutions at any given time. The central component of a paradigm is its current theoretical system. The most fruitful theoretical systems appear to be those that are relatively untested but seem to hold promise for establishing the relationship between the various phenomena of concern. These relatively untested theoretical systems provide an outline of the scientist's task. Or, as Kuhn would say, a paradigm outlines "puzzles to be solved."

The field of study of an academic discipline has some generally accepted or traditional boundaries. However, these boundaries may contract or expand, depending on the current paramount theoretical system of the discipline. Although there are commonly accepted principles of scientific inquiry, the theoretical system of a paradigm determines to some extent acceptable research methodology. For example, a particular theoretical system may dictate the nature and size of the sample, instruments for collecting data, and appropriate statistical analysis of the data collected.

A paradigm is somewhat more than a theoretical system and the process of formulating hypotheses and testing the validity of that system. It provides a sense of unity to the discipline. A paradigm facilitates communication and generates a spirit of camaraderie among members of a discipline.

The paradigm of a discipline may change over time, usually when data do not support the theoretical system or newly discovered phenomena cannot be accounted for in the context of the present theoretical system. This change may be revolutionary, leading to the formation of a new paradigm, or evolutionary, leading to periodic alterations in and refinements of the paradigm (87).

The major difficulty of using the concept of paradigm as a structure for occupational therapy is that occupational therapy is not an academic discipline; it is a profession. The concept of paradigm was formulated to describe and give structure to an academic discipline, not to a profession.

Clarification of the difference between an academic discipline and a profession may be useful at this point (33,69,82,107). The primary function of an academic discipline is the *creation of knowledge*: identifying common elements among varied phenomena, finding relationships between concepts, developing and testing theory. Society may or may not elect to use this knowledge now or in the future. The theoretical foundation of an academic discipline is, for the most part, derived from the various theories of the discipline itself. Occasionally theories or parts of theories from other disciplines may be incorporated into the theoretical system of a discipline, but this is a rather rare occurrence. However, new or hybrid disciplines may be created out of a combination of two or more disciplines (20,147,156). For example, social psychology and astrophysics are hybrid disciplines that formed their own theoretical foundation and, thus, paradigm and became fairly autonomous from their parent disciplines.

In contrast, the primary function of a profession is the *application of knowledge*. A profession is recognized by society because it provides services (based upon theoretical knowledge) that the society believes it needs to maintain its present and future well-being. A profession works with members of society to enhance their personal and social health, comfort, and prosperity. The theoretical foundation of a profession is for the most part derived from theories generated by the various disciplines. Only a small portion of a profession's theoretical foundation is developed by its own members (147).

The difference between an academic discipline and a profession can perhaps be clarified by examination of basic educational preparation and how the majority of members of a discipline and a profession spend their time. Preparation of an individual for entry into a discipline is characterized by study of the discipline's current theoretical system and the development of skills in research and theory building. Preparation of an individual for entry into a profession is characterized by study of the profession's theoretical foundation and how various theories are applied in day-to-day interactions with others. If a member of a discipline wishes to engage in application of knowledge or if a member of a profession wishes to engage in additional scientific pursuits, more advanced education is usually necessary. Thus, for example, a chemist who is interested in applying her knowledge may need to work toward a degree in chemical engineering; a nurse who is concerned with studying the effects of various nursing procedures may enter a doctoral degree program in nursing that emphasizes the development of research skills (42,46,53,59,107,141,162).

In regard to how the majority of the members of a discipline and a profession spend their time: If most scientists deserted their laboratories and computers, there would be a rapid and marked decrease in the fund of knowledge available to society. If most practitioners decided to engage in scientific pursuits, the needs of society would not be served.

With this short digression, the concept of paradigm provides a fairly good structure for understanding the nature of a discipline. A paradigm's focal point is the testing of a theoretical system which will enhance the general fund of knowledge available to mankind. The concept of paradigm, however, does not provide a suitable structure for a profession. It is not addressed to the application of knowledge. As defined by Kuhn, a paradigm includes neither a statement of philosophical assumptions nor an ethical code. Furthermore, there seems to be no place for a description of the nature of and principles for sequencing the various aspects of practice or a delineation of a profession's legitimate tools.

The concept of paradigm may be useful in further organization and study of the theoretical foundation of occupational therapy. But the theoretical foundation is only one component of a profession; it can neither stand alone nor provide adequate definition. Thus, the concept of paradigm does not seem to facilitate understanding of the generic, holistic nature of occupational therapy.

Section III
Exploration of Frames of Reference

12/ *Definition of Frames of Reference*

The model of a profession defines and delineates the broad outlines of a profession as it is understood by the profession and by society. Frames of reference further delineate a particular area or aspect of a profession and, as such, are the link between the profession's model and practice (52).

The concept "frame of reference" was occasionally used in the occupational therapy literature prior to 1968, but the term was never defined. It appears to have been used in the traditional dictionary sense of "a structure of concepts, values, customs, views, etc., by means of which an individual or group perceives or evaluates data, communicates ideas and regulates behavior" (152, p. 563). The term was defined in the occupational therapy literature in 1968 in a more specific and narrow manner.

As used in this text, a frame of reference is a set of interrelated internally consistent concepts, definitions, and postulates that provide a systematic description of and prescription for a practitioner's interaction within a particular aspect of a profession's domain of concern (108).

Again some clarification of terminology is in order. "A set of interrelated and internally consistent..." refers to the idea that all concepts, definitions, and postulates within a given frame of reference must be congruent one with the other. The theoretical base of a given frame of reference is often formulated by using components or elements from a number of different theoretical systems. Parts of a theory sometimes do not mesh easily with parts taken from other theories. Individuals, then, who formulate a frame of reference must take care that all of the components of various theories being utilized fit together in a logical and concise manner.

129

"Provide a systematic description of and prescription for a practitioner's interaction..." refers to two functions of a frame of reference. The first function is descriptive and relates to the actual practice of practitioners using a given frame of reference. A frame of reference in this sense is essentially a "word picture" of a practitioner's interactions in the evaluation and intervention process. The second function of a frame of reference is prescriptive in that it provides directions as to how a practitioner may interact in the evaluation and intervention process. Thus frames of reference provide information for the student relative to ways of interacting with clients. These same directions are, of course, also provided for the practitioner who wishes to use a new frame of reference. Frames of reference as prescriptive are not recipes; they provide guidelines for practice only.

"Domain of concern" as used in the above definition of frames of reference refers to a limited aspect of a profession's domain of concern. In occupational therapy a frame of reference may be concerned with only one performance component as exemplified in Ayers' (10) frame of reference regarding the sensory integrative skill of children. A frame of reference may, on the other hand, be concerned with more than one performance component. This is evident in analytic frames of reference, which tend to focus on cognitive and psychological function (47). Finally, frames of reference may be primarily concerned with one or more of the occupational performances. The "occupational behavior" frame of reference, for example, is concerned with all of the occupational therapy performances (25,29,41,77,78,127,129, 130). The domain of concern of a particular frame of reference tends, however, to be narrow and addressed to one area of practice.

The frames of reference of a profession are deduced from the model of the profession. In other words, the theoretical base of a frame of reference draws on various systems that are part of the theoretical foundation of the profession. The function-dysfunction continuums are an elaboration of one or more aspects of the profession's collective domain of concern. The tools suggested in a frame of reference consist of one or more of the tools considered legitimate by the profession. Frames of reference that are not deduced from a profession's model are considered to be, at best, irregular and eccentric. Individuals who use frames of reference that deviate significantly from the parameters of the profession's model are usually subject to formal or informal sanctions by the profession.

In the process of intervention with a client, more than one frame of reference is often used to guide practice. This is particularly true when the individual has multiple problems or areas of dysfunction. For example, one is likely to use several different frames of reference simultaneously to deal with the physical, psychological, and social sequelae of a severely burned client. No one frame of reference in occupational therapy provides guidelines for minimizing the deforming potential of scar tissue, assisting the individual to adjust to a serious alteration in physical appearance, and dealing with family members' reactions to touching and being with the client.

Professions have many different frames of reference that provide guidelines for dealing with various aspects of the profession's domain of concern. Professions also frequently have more than one frame of reference for dealing with the same area of practice. Two examples, one from medicine and one from education, may help to illustrate this phenomenon: Some psychiatrists prescribe medication to minimize a depressive reaction whereas others prescribe verbal psychotherapy. Some elementary school teachers believe that an open classroom is the best environment for developing skills in reading and writing; others favor a more structured environment.

Different frames of reference addressed to the same area of practice are often not compatible. For example, in occupational therapy one might use an analytic frame of reference as the basis for intervention in the area of psychosocial dysfunction. Or one might use a frame of reference based on the Skinnerian theory of operant conditioning as the basis for intervention in the same area. Different frames of reference addressed to the same area of practice may cause conflict within a profession. However, this is not to be viewed as detrimental to the profession or a sign of hopeless confusion. Such conflict enhances the vitality of a profession and assists in the clarification of ideas.

A practitioner's selection of a particular frame of reference is based on many factors. The setting of intervention and the nature of the client population are significant factors. However, the practitioner's area of expertise, life view, and inclinations are also of great importance in the selection of a frame of reference.

In the past, the concept of frame of reference has been used to give structure to that part of evaluation and intervention which is concerned with the change process only. In other words, frames of reference have not been addressed to prevention, maintenance, management, or meeting health needs. This has probably occurred because the structure of frames of reference was originally designed to deal only with the change process. However, with some minor alteration in the component parts of frames of reference, the concept is able to be used to structure all aspects of evaluation and intervention. These minor alterations are reflected in the next chapter.

The relationship between a profession's model and its various frames of reference is discussed in Chapter 15. Suffice it to say at this point that a model provides boundaries for and gives general direction to a profession as a whole. A frame of reference provides guidelines in the immediacy of daily interactions with clients.

13/ *Structure of Frames of Reference*

This chapter describes the structure of frames of reference. Particular frames of reference are mentioned in an illustrative manner only. It is not the purpose of this text to explore the content of various frames of reference in occupational therapy. Just as one may speak of the structure of theory or of professional models regardless of content, so also can one speak of the structure of a frame of reference without study of content.

In outline form, then, the structure of a frame of reference is made up of:

1. A statement of the theoretical base;
2. Delineation of function-dysfunction continuums;
3. A listing of behaviors indicative of function and dysfunction;
4. Postulates regarding intervention.

THEORETICAL BASE

The theoretical base of a frame of reference delineates the concepts and their definition and postulates which are necessary for an adequate description of and rationale for the type of intervention suggested by the frame of reference in its totality. It is referred to as the *base* of a frame of reference because it identifies the parameters of the frame of reference and serves as the matrix from which all other parts of the frame of reference are deduced. The type of content included in a theoretical base varies somewhat depending on the aspect of human function to which the frame of reference is addressed or the type of evaluation and intervention for which it is to serve as a guide.

In general terms, the theoretical base describes the nature of the area of human function of concern in the frame of reference and the effect of the human and nonhuman environment on that area of human function. More specifically, normal development and developmental deviations are described; factors inherent to an individual and external environmental factors that influence normal and deviant development are delineated; interactions with the human and nonhuman environment that are believed to alter deficits in the direction of function are defined. For example, if a frame of reference is addressed to the area of self-concept, the theoretical base includes a description of how an individual acquires an accurate self-concept through interaction with the human and nonhuman environment, how an individual maintains a particular self-concept, and how an individual develops an inaccurate self-concept. Further, the theoretical base outlines in general terms how interaction with the environment leads to alteration of an inaccurate self-concept.

A theoretical base may be formulated from one theoretical system, or concepts, definitions, and postulates may be drawn from several different theoretical systems. The latter is more often the case because many theories important to the practice of occupational therapy are static. A static theory describes relationships between various phenomena but does not account for the factor of change or alteration. Examples of static theories are human anatomy, which describes the structures of the body and their relationship one to the other, and Piaget's theory of cognition, which describes various stages of cognitive development (51,120). Human anatomy describes the potential for movement of the body, but it does not describe how body parts are coordinated in actual movement. Piaget's theory of cognition delineates stages of cognitive development, but it does not say how an individual moves from one stage of development to another. In contrast, dynamic theories deal with the issues of change, movement, alteration, maintenance, and the like. Examples of dynamic theories are kinesiology, which is the study of human movement, and learning theories, which attempt to account for a relatively permanent change in behavior over a period of time.

If a static theory is used as part of a frame of reference, a dynamic theory of one sort or another must also be used. The theoretical base of a frame of reference concerned with neuromotor function, for example, would most likely include concepts, definitions, and postulates from both anatomy and kinesiology. The theoretical base of a frame of reference concerned with cognition may use Piaget's theory of stages of cognitive development but would also need to include at least some aspects of a learning theory in order to describe movement from one stage of development to another. Some theories are both static and dynamic. Sullivan's (153) theory of psychosocial development, for example, describes both stages of development and the environmental factors that facilitate movement from one stage of development to another. Thus, the theoretical base of a frame of reference concerned with psychosocial development may be drawn entirely from Sullivanian theory.

A theoretical base may or may not deal with "cause," or antecedent events believed to be directly related to dysfunction. If the elaboration of antecedent events contributes to an understanding of evaluation or intervention relative to dysfunction, then a description of these events should be part of the theoretical base. If antecedent events are irrelevant to evaluation and intervention, then it is unnecessary and at times confusing to describe these events in the theoretical base. Dysfunction or deficit may arise from and be maintained by any number of known and unknown factors that have influenced the individual. If these factors are organic in nature and still amenable to alteration through surgical or pharmacological intervention, then the frame of reference is within the domain of medicine, not occupational therapy. If the factors considered to be antecedent to dysfunction are located in the individual's past history, they are not amenable to change. Therefore, they are not included in a frame of reference. If the antecedent factors leading to dysfunction are considered to be currently operating in the individual's present environment, then dysfunction is located in the environment and not the individual. For example, a child may have a "school phobia" because the parents do not really want the child to move out of a position of dependency on the home. Although indeed the child might need some assistance, the frame of reference that deals with this issue most directly is addressed to the dysfunction of the parents, not that of the child.

In summary, the theoretical base of a frame of reference describes the area(s) of human function of concern in the frame of reference, factors that influence normal and deviant development, and interactions with the human and nonhuman environment believed to alter deficits in the direction of function. Antecedent events or current factors that influence dysfunction are included in the theoretical base of a frame of reference only to the extent to which they facilitate an understanding of the evaluation and intervention process.

FUNCTION-DYSFUNCTION CONTINUUMS

A function-dysfunction continuum is a label that identifies one area of human function. An individual's degree of function is classified on a range from the total inability to engage in a particular function to complete mastery of that function. Some examples of function-dysfunction continuums are given below:

Visual form and space perception

Inability to distinguish various forms and their orientation in space ←————→ Age-appropriate skill in distinguishing forms and their orientation in space

Muscle strength

No evidence of muscle contraction ←————→ Ability to move a body part against heavy resistance

Group interaction skill

Inability to participate in a parallel group ←————→ Ability to participate in a mature group

The concept "continuum" is important in understanding this part of the structure of a frame of reference. The term *continuum* was chosen to indicate that there is essentially no break or line of demarcation between that which is considered function and that which is considered dysfunction. Function is considered to be relative to age, cultural background, and present environment. For example, an adolescent in our society is not expected to be self-supporting; an individual of 25 years of age is expected in most cases to be self-supporting. The individual who cannot sew on a button or mend a ripped seam is not considered to be in a state of dysfunction in the area of self-care if there is someone in the environment who is willing and able to sew on a button or mend a ripped seam for the individual. Function-dysfunction then is viewed as an uninterrupted line and relative to the life circumstances of a particular individual.

The function-dysfunction continuums outlined in a frame of reference are deduced from the theoretical base of a frame of reference. In the theoretical base, function and dysfunction are described in general terms. However, the nature of function and dysfunction is made more specific in this portion of a frame of reference. For example, in the theoretical base, "task skills" might be defined as the collection of abilities which an individual must have in order to carry out a relatively complex task. In the section devoted to delineating function-dysfunction continuums, the general category of task skill may be broken down into its component parts. Function-dysfunction continuums might then be:

> the ability to concentrate;
> the ability to follow illustrated, written, and verbal directions;
> the ability to solve problems within the context of a task;
> the ability to give appropriate attention to detail;
> and so on.

Function-dysfunction continuums, then, are deduced from the theoretical base and more specifically enumerated in the section on function-dysfunction continuums.

A frame of reference may have one or several function-dysfunction continuums. Most frames of reference have more than one continuum, but no particular number is appropriate. The criterion for judging numerical adequacy is whether the continuums identify all of the component parts of the human function(s) to which the frame of reference is addressed.

If there is more than one continuum in a frame of reference, these continuums should be relatively mutually exclusive and stated on the same conceptual level. An example of two relatively mutually exclusive continuums is eye-hand coordination and the capacity to engage in intimate relations. The word *relatively* is emphasized here because the individual is a holistic being. One identifies areas of function while recognizing that at the level of total integration each function influences the adequacy or inadequacy of all other functions.

Each function-dysfunction continuum must be stated on the same conceptual level. For example, it is better to identify dimensions such as work habits, interpersonal skills, and coordination as function-dysfunction continuums in a given frame of reference than to identify dimensions such as reality testing, ego strength, and impulse control. Work habits, interpersonal skills, and coordination are fairly equal relative to conceptual level. Reality testing, ego strength, and impulse control are not on the same conceptual level; reality testing and impulse control are considered to be ego functions. Function-dysfunction continuums which are relatively mutually exclusive and stated on the same conceptual level facilitate the process of evaluation and intervention.

BEHAVIOR INDICATIVE OF FUNCTION OR DYSFUNCTION

In addition to naming or labeling the function-dysfunction continuum, a frame of reference also provides operational definitions or behavior indicative of function and dysfunction relative to the various continuums stated. For example, behaviors indicative of function on the continuum "awareness of body parts and their relationship" are likely to be:

1. the ability to identify individual fingers when they have been touched by an examiner (with vision occluded);
2. the ability to name the various body parts;
3. the ability to state the spatial relationship between various body parts; and
4. the ability to identify various positions of body parts without the aid of vision.

In contrast, behavior indicative of dysfunction on the continuum of "trust in one's fellow man" might be:

1. expresses fear of others;
2. acts shy and fearful of the therapist;
3. makes derogatory comments about others;
4. has few friends;
5. demonstrates difficulty in getting along with others;
6. is suspicious of others' intentions.

In order to facilitate evaluation, behavior indicative of function and dysfunction is outlined in the most specific way possible. The degree of specificity often depends on the continuum under consideration. Behavior indicative of function or dysfunction tends to be more specific in those frames of reference which are addressed, for example, to neuromotor function or sensory integration.

Behaviors indicative of function-dysfunction may be provided in a frame of reference relative only to function or to dysfunction. In such a case the absence of behaviors indicative of function indicates dysfunction and conversely the absence of behaviors indicative of dysfunction indicates function. Some frames of reference provide a listing of both behaviors indicative of function and behaviors indicative of dysfunction.

In most frames of reference one behavior alone is not sufficient to identify either function or dysfunction. The presence or absence of a gestalt of behaviors serves best to identify function or dysfunction. In that function-dysfunction continuums are rarely entirely mutually exclusive, a particular behavior indicative of function or dysfunction may be listed under two or more continuums. For example, "minimal attention to personal hygiene or dress" may be stated as being indicative of negative feelings about one's self, disregard for the standards set by society, or lack of skill in the area of self-care. Usually only by awareness of the gestalt of behaviors indicative of function or dysfunction is one able to assess specific areas of function or dysfunction.

What is identified as dysfunction in one frame of reference may be described as behavior indicative of dysfunction in another frame of reference. For example, in one frame of reference anxiety regarding travel may be identified as a behavior indicative of unmet security needs. In another frame of reference anxiety regarding travel may be identified simply as an area of dysfunction. The goal of intervention in the former frame of reference may be to assist the client in identifying unconscious ideas relative to feelings of insecurity. The goal of intervention relative to the latter frame of reference would be to assist the client in learning how to travel without experiencing anxiety. What is dysfunction as opposed to behavior indicative of dysfunction varies from one frame of reference to another. The intervention process is directed toward minimizing or eliminating dysfunction with the assumption that behavior indicative of dysfunction will gradually cease to be a part of the individual's repertoire of behavior as the individual moves toward a state of function.

Behavior indicative of function and dysfunction forms the basis for evaluation, as described in Chapter 11 in the section on activity and analysis and synthesis. In some frames of reference, however, specific evaluative techniques are suggested. Ideally, these techniques are described in such a manner that they can be duplicated by any practitioner to elicit the desired behavior. The way in which the elicited behavior or findings are to be interpreted should also be provided. This, it must be emphasized, is the ideal. Unfortunately, there are few standardized evaluation procedures in occupational therapy. A standardized evaluation procedure is comprised of empirically selected materials and activities, specific directions for use, acceptable levels of reliability, and validity and norms based on adequate sample size and appropriate population (18,75,113,121,144,147,149).

In the above definition of standardized evaluation procedures, "empirical" refers to the selection of materials and activities based on factual and systematic investigation. "Specific directions for use" refers to how the therapist will behave, the directions to be given, the sequence of the evaluation procedure, and time limitations if any. "Reliability" is the degree of dependability, stability, and accuracy of an evaluation procedure. It is essentially concerned with the question of whether similar behavior would be observed if an individual were involved in a given evaluative procedure repeatedly at several different times. Although small changes in behavior might be evident, reliable evaluation procedures are designed to identify basic, persistent patterns of behavior. If an evaluation procedure is not reliable, the practitioner is unable to make a statement about the client's state of function or dysfunction with any degree of dependability or confidence in that statement. "Validity" refers to whether the evaluation procedure is assessing what is stated that the procedure is supposed to be able to assess. To clarify, if a particular evaluation procedure is designed to assess whether an individual has the ability to form abstract concepts, the scoring and interpretation of the behavior exhibited during the procedure must lead to accurate statements about the individual's ability to form abstract concepts in a variety of situations unrelated to the evaluation setting. "Norms" are a statement, often in tabular form, of a single performance or a range of performances similar to the usual performance of a given group of individuals. Norms are determined by administering a particular evaluation procedure to a large number of individuals who are included in a particular category, e.g., college sophomores, 8-year-old girls, or individuals who live in one of the large urban centers on the eastern coast of the United States.

There are a few quasi-standardized evaluation procedures outlined in various occupational therapy frames of reference; these are addressed primarily to the performance components of sensory integration and neuromuscular function. Most of the evaluation procedures one finds in frames of reference for occupational therapy are approximately midway between subjective and objective. A subjective evaluative procedure is one in which there are no standards or criteria for scoring or interpreting findings. An objective evaluative procedure eliminates, as far as possible, the influence of the examiner's bias or opinion and can be scored or interpreted by the application of simple rules requiring a minimum of judgment. Evaluative procedures which are midway between subjective and objective have some broad criterion for scoring or interpretation; however, it is also necessary to use a good deal of subjective professional judgment.

In some professions, standardized evaluative procedures are seen as the factor that will allow the profession to be recognized as equal with other professions. This is highly questionable. Many areas of human function cannot be measured by standardized tests and procedures. Even in those professions that have been the bastion of standardized testing such as psychology and education, doubts have been raised as to the validity of many standardized tests. It is, indeed, desirable to have evaluative tools and procedures which are as objective as possible. But professional interpretation and judgment are a significant part of any evaluation procedure.

POSTULATES REGARDING INTERVENTION

Postulates regarding intervention are descriptive or prescriptive statements, deduced from the theoretical base, which state the principles by which prevention of dysfunction occurs, function is maintained, interfering behavior is managed, an individual is assisted in moving from a state of dysfunction to a state of function, or health needs are met. Postulates regarding intervention state the nature, quality, quantity, and sequence of interactions with the human and nonhuman environments which are believed to facilitate intervention. Postulates regarding intervention also state relationships that guide the practitioner in selection of immediate and long-term goals, the step-by-step progression of intervention in each area of dysfunction, and the postulates applicable during each stage of intervention. The following are examples of postulates regarding intervention:

1. Fine motor planning is enhanced by engaging in purposeful activities that require increasingly more precise and complex planning for their proper execution.
2. The ability to trust another human being is acquired through extensive interaction between two persons in which one individual receives consistent and relatively immediate need satisfaction, is not required to give any reciprocal satisfaction, and is free to engage in any behavior which is not destructive to the self or others.

3. Adaptive behavior is increased through the judicious use of positive and differential reinforcement in conjunction with the process of shaping and building chains of performance.

By convention, postulates regarding intervention are stated in a specific form. The beginning phrase or stem of a postulate identifies the area of function with which the postulate is concerned. Thus a postulate such as "purposeful motor activity enhances the integration of sensory stimuli" is poorly stated because the area of function is identified at the end of the postulate. This convention was developed simply because a statement of function at the beginning of a postulate makes it easier for the reader to comprehend. In a postulate regarding intervention, the area of function-dysfunction is usually stated in the positive. For example, "the frequency of secondary process thinking is increased by..." is more acceptable than "the frequency of primary process thinking is decreased by...." This convention is probably based on the belief of most practitioners that the development of adaptive behavior is far more important than simply diminishing maladaptive behavior or dysfunctional behavior.

In addition, and perhaps far more important, a postulate regarding intervention is addressed to the nature of the external environment and not what the client will somehow accomplish in an undefined manner. An example of a postulate that describes the external environment is "A more accurate self-concept is acquired through feedback from others regarding the individual's capacity to engage in specific activities." An example of a postulate addressed to what the client will do is "A more accurate self-concept is acquired through an understanding of one's assets and limitations." The point to be made is that postulates regarding intervention are articulated to guide the therapist in synthesizing or designing activities that will facilitate the development of function. The second postulate stated above does not provide such guidance.

A frame of reference never predicts what a client will do when involved in an intervention process. Thus postulates regarding intervention never allude to the behavior of a client. Phrases such as "... is enhanced through the opportunity to interact..." or "... is facilitated by participation in..." are used deliberately. The therapist is only able to design appropriate activities and encourage the client to participate in these activities. The client must decide whether movement toward function is desirable and then engage in the work of learning.

Postulates regarding intervention are concerned with interaction relative to the human and the nonhuman environments. Thus, in designing activities, the occupational therapist considers his interpersonal interactions with the client, an interaction process relative to the nonhuman environment, and the interplay between the two. The occupational therapist never considers interpersonal relationships outside of the context of the nonhuman environment or the nonhuman environment outside of the context of interpersonal relationships. All activities then have an interpersonal component and a component of interaction with the nonhuman environment.

Postulates regarding intervention may be general or specific. A general postulate applies to a number of or all areas of dysfunction identified in a particular frame of reference. A specific postulate regarding intervention applies to one area of dysfunction identified in a particular frame of reference. The following examples illustrate these two types of postulates:

1. Perception in a given sensory system is enhanced by general sensory stimulation which requires an adaptive motor response. The stimuli must be sufficiently intense to be received by the central nervous system yet not cause overarousal.
2. Development of ocular control is facilitated by encouraging the client to focus on stationary and moving objects both within a central field of vision and peripheral to the central field of vision.

The first postulate relates to the integration of the sensory system regardless of the particular sensory stimuli under consideration. The second postulate is concerned with ocular control, only one aspect of sensory integration.

The types of postulates contained within a given frame of reference are relatively unimportant. What is important is that the postulates are deduced from the theoretical base and adequately describe or prescribe the process of intervention relative to the continuums to which the frame of reference is addressed.

CONCLUSION

In summary, the structure of a frame of reference consists of a theoretical base, function-dysfunction continuums, behavior indicative of function and dysfunction, and postulates regarding intervention. There are a variety of different frames of reference in occupational therapy. This variety provides for professional viability and choices on the part of practitioners. The common structure of frames of reference facilitates communication. Even in the midst of heated debate, there is at least a shared language.

14/ *Types of Frames of Reference*

The structure of a frame of reference can be used to organize all aspects of evaluation and intervention—prevention, maintenance management, the change process, and meeting health needs. However, at this time, published frames of reference are only or primarily addressed to the change process. This may be the case because the change process is often seen as being the most prestigious aspect of the occupational therapy process. It also tends to be the most difficult area to explain to others. But, regardless of the reason, there are no published frames of reference specifically addressed to prevention, maintenance, management, and meeting health needs.

Thus, in this chapter frames of reference relative to the change process only are discussed. The purpose of this chapter is to present a brief taxonomy of the various frames of reference currently available. Admittedly, not all of the frames of reference fall easily into one specific category. In placing a particular frame of reference in a specific category, the major criterion used was the general orientation of the frame of reference. Minor variations within a frame of reference that might support placing it in another category were essentially ignored. After studying the various frames of reference, the reader may well decide that one or several should be placed in a different category or that for greater accuracy additional categories need to be developed. However, for the purpose of this text, frames of reference addressed to the change process are placed in three different categories: analytical, developmental, and acquisitional.

ANALYTICAL FRAMES OF REFERENCE

Analytical frames of reference are addressed to the performance components of cognitive function, psychological function, and social interaction

Frames of reference other than analytical are also addressed to these performance components; but these are the only performance components considered in analytical frames of reference.

Analytical frames of reference are based on two major assumptions. The first is that mature behavior is developed, restored, or enhanced by bringing symptom-producing unconscious conflicts to consciousness and integrating this previously unconscious content with conscious content. The second assumption is that generalized adaptive behavior, whether new or previously learned, will emerge with the integration of unconscious and conscious content (25,52).

The theoretical base of an analytic frame of reference describes the individual as continually striving for need fulfillment, expression of primitive impulses, and control of inherent drives. In the usual course of events, the individual learns how to meet needs, express impulses, and control drives in a manner both satisfying to the self and acceptable within the norms of the individual's cultural group. This learning occurs through interaction in an environment that recognizes the individual's needs, drives, and impulses and provides a variety of learning experiences to assist the individual in controlling their expression. Eventually, the individual accepts the norms of his or her cultural group: these norms become a part of the individual's value system. This process occurs because, through acceptance of the norms of one's cultural group, the individual is accepted as a full-fledged member of the group and receives all of the rewards commensurate with such membership.

However, this process sometimes does not occur in the manner outlined above for many reasons that are outside of the parameters of this text. Suffice it to say that, for whatever reason, the individual may experience needs, drives, and impulses as being in conflict with each other, with the reality of the environment, or with the individual's value system.

Such conflictual experiences tend to arouse anxiety, which in turn leads to repression of the conflict. The individual either pushes these conflicts out of consciousness or does not allow the affect, ideas, and desires related to the conflictual experience to become conscious. This repressed information, however, still tends to influence behavior. Without knowledge of the nature of an individual's unconscious conflicts, the behavior of the individual may seem somewhat irrational to the individual and to an observer. However, according to psychoanalytic theory, this behavior is considered to follow certain principles. *Psychodynamics* is the term used to designate the relationship and study of the relationship between unconscious conflict and "irrational" behavior. Thus using a particular theory of psychodynamics an expert, given a set of irrational behaviors, can fairly accurately predict the nature of unconscious conflict. Conversely, with knowledge of the unconscious conflict the expert is able to predict, with some degree of accuracy, the individual's behavior. It is important to note, however, that our understanding of psychodynamics is limited and that there are several different theories of psychodynamics. Practitioners who use an analytic frame of reference are more involved in exploration of the mysteries of the human mind and behavior than in the application of an exact science.

Symptom-producing unconscious conflict is considered to be dysfunction in analytic frames of reference. These conflicts tend to center around such issues as love, hate, aggression, sexuality, autonomy, trust, feelings of inadequacy, and death.

Behavior indicative of dysfunction is any behavior that cannot be explained given the realities of the situation or environment. More specifically the nature of unconscious conflict is determined through study and understanding of the individual's past history, current behavior, and symbolic communication.

Change takes place through bringing symptom-producing unconscious content to consciousness. This is accomplished by the therapist being supportive and accepting and remaining a fairly unknown entity to the client The latter encourages the client to respond to the therapist in a manner similar to the way in which the client responded to one or more significant individuals in the client's past life experience. This phenomenon, referred to as transference, allows the client and therapist to become aware of past important interpersonal relationships that may have been repressed by the client. One of the major vehicles for bringing unconscious content to consciousness is the use of symbols. These may be symbols produced in dream or through working with unstructured media such as clay or finger paint When unstructured media are used, both the process and the product are explored. Symbols are studied relative to their possible universal, cultural and personal meanings. The possible meanings of transference behavior and symbols are shared by the client and the therapist in order to understand them within the context of the client's unique life experience. This process is referred to as interpretation. Ideally, interpretation is followed by insight on the part of the client. Insight is a cognitive or conscious understanding of the meaning and purpose of one's behavior. The final step is referred to as working through. This is the process of facing and dealing with the same, now conscious conflict, over and over again in daily life until the conflict is resolved and no longer influences behavior. It is assumed that the individual is able to independently continue toward self-actualization when symptom-producing unconscious content is integrated with conscious content.

The frames of reference in occupational therapy that appear to be analytic in nature are the Fidlers' orientation to intervention as exemplified in *Occupational Therapy: A Communication Process in Psychiatry* (47) and Mosey's "Object Relation Analysis" (108).

DEVELOPMENTAL FRAMES OF REFERENCE

Developmental frames of reference may be addressed to one or more of the performance components or occupational performances. They may be unidimensional, dealing with only one area of function, or they may be multidimensional, dealing with several areas of function.

Developmental frames of reference are based on several assumptions. The first is that the individual progresses through specific stages of development in various areas of human function. In each stage the individual's behavior or skills are qualitatively different than they are relative to a past or future stage in that particular area. "Qualitatively different" refers to the idea that something new is added at each stage. This addition does not mean refinement of a skill—as, for example, an increase in coordination, but something entirely new added to the individual's repertoire of behavior. Behavior from a previous stage is usually integrated with the new emerging stage. An appropriate analogy for developmental frames of reference is to think of each area of function as a stairway with each step representing a specific stage of maturation.

In multidimensional developmental frames of reference, each area of function is considered to be interdependent with the other areas of function specified in the frame of reference. Thus deficits or lack of age-specific stage development in one area of function will inhibit appropriate growth in other areas of function. Normal development in various areas of function tends to be naturally uneven for any given individual. However, if development in one or more areas lags too far behind that in other areas, the individual is likely to have problems in the total developmental process.

The concept of splinter skills is important in developmental frames of reference. The individual may appear to be at a particular stage of development in one area yet appear not to have acquired the underlying stage-specific skills. Splinter skills are stage-specific behaviors that have been learned by rote, in a mechanical or nonintegrated manner. Behavior so learned takes considerable energy to maintain and is the first behavior to be lost from the individual's repertoire in times of stress. Individuals who have acquired splinter skills may appear to be able to interact quite effectively in the community. However, in the face of stressful situations, their behavior reverts to a far less mature stage of development. Behavior tends to revert to those stages of development that have been acquired in an integrated manner. When a developmental frame of reference is used, the teaching of splinter skills is avoided and stage-by-stage learning of skills is emphasized.

The cause of lack of age-appropriate skills is not considered to be of particular importance in developmental frames of reference. The individual's current status is important, regardless of whether a particular stage of development has ever been mastered, whether it was learned by rote, or whether it has been lost through neurological impairment.

Finally, it is assumed that interacting in an environment which simulates the usual optimal environment for the acquisition of a particular stage of development in a given area of human function will allow the individual to acquire the necessary behavior in an integrated manner. It is also assumed that the individual must go through all stages of development in a particular area in order to reach the appropriate age-specific level.

The theoretical base of developmental frames of reference describes the sequential stages of development of those areas of function addressed in the frame of reference. In addition, the theoretical base describes those factors in the environment, both human and nonhuman, which are believed to lead to movement from one stage of development to the next stage of development. The theoretical bases of developmental frames of reference vary depending on the areas of function of concern and the theories of human development being utilized.

Function-dysfunction continuums in a developmental frame of reference consist of specific areas of human function. Each component of the continuum is divided into various stages. The number of stages varies as does the life span taken into consideration. Most published developmental frames of reference begin with the initial stage of development of the areas of function addressed in the frame of reference. The last stages mentioned tend to be those reached by late childhood or middle adolescence. The age range identified is likely to be expanded as there are now several recent theories regarding human development through the adult years. In the outline of the continuums, the approximate chronological age for the normal acquisition of each stage is usually given.

Behavior indicative of function or dysfunction is a listing of specific behaviors an individual usually exhibits if he has or has not mastered a given stage of development. Thus behavior indicative of function or dysfunction is provided for each of the stages of development mentioned in the one or more continuums of the frame of reference. Behavior directly observed by the therapist and the client's recent behavior in the community are used as the basis for evaluation.

Postulates regarding change in a developmental frame of reference may be general or stage specific. General postulates state how learning occurs regardless of any particular stage or area of development. They are usually deduced from a theory or theories of learning outlined in the theoretical base of the frame of reference. Specific postulates state the type of environmental interaction which is believed to allow for movement from one given stage of development to the next stage of development. When specific postulates are used, there is a postulate regarding intervention for each stage of development.

The criteria for setting initial and long-term goals are similar in all developmental frames of reference. The change process is initiated in that area of function in which stage-specific learning is the most primitive. Acquisition of skill continues in that area through each sequentially more advanced stage until learning in that area is equal to learning in the area of function in which stage-specific learning is next most primitive. The change process in this area is then initiated. This sequence continues until all stages of development needed in the client's expected environment are mastered or until it appears that the individual is unable to move to more advanced stages of development.

The frames of reference in occupational therapy which appear to be developmental in nature are Reilly's frame of reference as described in *Play as Exploratory Learning* (131); "Occupational Behavior" (25,29,41,77); the frames of reference outlined by Banus (12) and Llorens (91,92); sensory integration as described by Ayres (10,11) and King (80); the neurodevelopmental approaches of Rood, Bobath, and Brunnstrom (154); proprioceptive neuromuscular facilitation (154); and "Recapitulation of Ontogenesis" as described by Mosey (108).

ACQUISITIONAL FRAMES OF REFERENCE

Acquisitional frames of reference may be addressed to one or more of the performance components or occupational performances. Similar to developmental frames of reference, they may be unidimensional or multidimensional.

Acquisitional frames of reference are based on the assumption that the areas of function included in the frame of reference are non-stage specific, quantitatively different, and independent one from the other. *Non-stage specific* refers to the fact that there are no identifiable stages of development for a particular area of function. *Quantitative difference* refers to the assumption that a given skill only increases or becomes more refined over time. An example of the difference between qualitative and quantitative change may be useful. It appears that the original acquisition of language is qualitative in nature. The child acquires the parts of speech (nouns, verbs, adjectives, etc.) step by step. At each step a new part of speech is added to the child's repertoire. After all the parts of speech have been learned, acquisition of additional language skill appears to be quantitative. There is a steady increase in vocabulary but no new parts of speech are added to the child's repertoire. Finally, the various areas of function in an acquisitional frame of reference, in contrast to those in a developmental frame of reference, are considered to be independent of each other. Lack of learning in one area is not considered to impede learning in other areas of function.

In acquisitional frames of reference little attention is given to the reasons why an individual has not acquired a particular skill. This information is not considered important in designing an appropriate intervention process.

The theoretical base of an acquisitional frame of reference is usually derived from one or more theories of learning and/or the theories which serve as the foundation of activity groups. The general skills or behaviors necessary for participation in the community are outlined. However, there is no concern about when these skills are usually acquired in the normal developmental process.

The function-dysfunction continuums of an acquisitional frame of reference tend to be fairly specific. In other words, the focus is on concrete skills as opposed to a more abstract cluster of stage-specific skills typical of developmental frames of reference.

Behaviors indicative of function and dysfunction in an acquisition frame of reference also tend to be specific. Evaluation focuses on the question of whether an individual has certain skills in her current repertoire of behavior and how frequently these skills are used in interactions within the community. Evaluation is primarily oriented to the client's current repertoire of behavior rather than past capacities or abilities. In addition, the evaluation process may also involve assessment of environmental factors that appear to be responsible for the individual's present repertoire and frequency of particular types of behavior.

The postulates regarding intervention in acquisitional frames of reference tend to be general in nature. In other words, the postulates are addressed to the acquisition of all of the continuums included in a particular frame of reference. Postulates are concerned with the ways one may assist a client to acquire or increase functional behavior. But postulates also may be concerned with ways within the context of the clinical setting to alter the client's environment within the community so that there is continued support for functional behavior.

The criteria for goal setting are less specific in acquisitional frames of reference than in developmental frames of reference. The criteria also vary from one acquisitional frame of reference to another. However, in general, the major criterion used is the most important or useful behavior for the client to acquire at that time. Ideally, the client and therapist together determine the most important behavior to be acquired.

The frames of reference in occupational therapy that appear to be acquisitional in nature are those based on the theory of operant conditioning (68,98,148,158), *Activities Therapy* as described by Mosey (111), and the biomechanical and rehabilitative frames of reference outlined by Trombly and Scott (154).

DIFFERENCES BETWEEN THE VARIOUS TYPES OF FRAMES OF REFERENCE

Some of the differences between acquisitional frames of reference and developmental frames of reference are mentioned in the above section. However, identification of additional differences between various types of frames of reference may be useful (52,108).

In analytic frames of reference the dysfunction of concern is unconscious conflict. Lack of skill development in various areas of human function is behavior indicative of dysfunction. The change process is directed toward resolving unconscious conflict. It is assumed that skills needed for productive interaction in the community will spontaneously be learned or re-learned after the resolution of unconscious conflict. Conversely, in developmental and acquisitional frames of reference, lack of skill development in various areas of human function is the dysfunction of concern. Unconscious conflict, if mentioned at all, is behavior indicative of dysfunction. The change process is directed toward acquiring skills in various areas of human function. It is assumed that unconscious conflict will disappear spontaneously with the acquisition of skills.

In analytic frames of reference, transference, the development of insight, and working through previously unconscious conflicts are considered paramount. These processes are not a part of developmental or acquisitional frames of reference. Transference is discouraged and the processes of insight and working through are not considered to be relevant. The concept of learning is not used in analytic frames of reference, whereas in developmental and acquisitional frames of reference it is usually an important component of the theoretical base and the postulates regarding intervention.

Some developmental frames of reference make considerable use of symbolic activities. However, these activities are used differently than they are in analytic frames of reference. In developmental frames of reference symbolic activities are used to assist the client in re-experiencing and mastering primitive stages of development, such as gratification of infantile needs. In analytic frames of reference the symbolic meaning of activities is explored to help the client to become aware of and integrate unconscious content.

Analytic frames of reference never provide for gratification of infantile needs. Acquisitional frames of reference are usually not concerned with the symbolic nature of purposeful activity.

The degree of awareness or consciousness required on the part of the client is different in analytic frames of reference as opposed to developmental frames of reference. In the former, various stages of the client's personal development may be discussed, explored, and in this way brought to conscious awareness. In the application of developmental frames of reference, the client is not requested to be aware of the symbolic nature of activities or of need gratification. The experience, not the conscious awareness of the experience, is considered important.

One of the major differences between developmental and acquisitional frames of reference is related to the assumptions regarding the acquisition of an appropriate level of skill in performance components and occupational performance. In developmental frames of reference these areas of function are considered to be stage specific, qualitatively different, and interdependent. In acquisitional frames of reference these areas of function are considered to be non-stage specific, quantitatively different, and independent.

In considering the three types of frames of reference and in outlining their differences no attempt has been made to indicate the superiority of any one. The various frames of reference in occupational therapy offer the practitioner a variety of choices in regard to selecting a guide for evaluation and intervention. Additional frames of reference will be formulated in the future. Previously formulated frames of reference will become obsolete. This is a normal process in any profession and a sign of healthy continued growth and development.

15/ Additional Comments Regarding Frames of Reference

To further clarify the nature of frames of reference, we will discuss in this chapter two areas: the relationship of frames of reference to theory and the relationship of frames of reference to the concept of model.

RELATIONSHIP TO THEORY

A frame of reference is not a theory. It is similar to theory in that it uses concepts, definitions, and postulates—the structural components of theory. A frame of reference is founded on or deduced from one or more theories or parts of several theories, as previously mentioned. However, a frame of reference differs from a theory in that it contains postulates or principles for guiding action.

A theory is descriptive. Its function is to predict relationships between a circumscribed set of events or phenomena. No action is implied or recommended. By way of illustration, typically theories of child development describe the maturation and growth of children from either conception or birth to the beginning of adolescence. No guidelines are provided for fostering maturation and growth. However, suggestions for child rearing are available in a variety of books. These suggestions are deduced from theories of child development. In this sense one may speak of various frames of reference for child rearing. Frames of reference are founded on theories, but the functions of theories and frames of reference are different. The function of theory is to predict; that of a frame of reference is to guide action.

Frames of reference, ideally, are based on theories that have been verified by considerable research. In actuality, this is not always the case. Frames of reference in occupational therapy are often based on embryonic theories that have been subjected to little empirical testing. Such frames of reference are utilized because without them either many clients would be deprived of at least some opportunity to develop skills necessary for community living or practitioners' interactions with clients would be guided only by intuition or a compassionate desire to serve mankind. Obviously, neither course of action is desirable or conducive to the development and maintenance of function. A practitioner is able to act only on the basis of currently available knowledge, fully recognizing the tremendous number of unknown factors inherent in the process.

RELATIONSHIP TO THE CONCEPT OF MODEL

The frames of reference of a profession and the model of a profession differ in three ways: magnitude, universality of acceptance, and degree of guidance.

In relation to magnitude, a model defines and gives boundaries to a profession. A particular frame of reference, on the other hand, defines and gives boundaries to a small aspect of the profession's domain of concern. An example from elementary education may be useful. The model for elementary education outlines the academic and social skills (among other skills) for which elementary school teachers are responsible. Frames of reference of elementary education provide guidelines for developing skills in the area of mathematics or for enhancing cooperation in and outside of the classroom. Models are broad in focus; frames of reference are limited and narrow in focus.

A model, as mentioned previously, is accepted almost universally by the profession and the society to which it is responsible. A given frame of reference is often accepted by only a limited number of practitioners within a profession. For example, in occupational therapy, only some practitioners accept King's frame of reference regarding sensory integration as an appropriate guide for intervention relative to clients diagnosed as schizophrenic. A few years ago there was considerable controversy over the use of frames of reference based on the theory of operant conditioning. A model, because it is more generally stated, tends to engender little disharmony.

Frames of reference, being more specific, often become the focus for considerable professional disagreement. However, such conflict also may lead to clarification of concepts and productive research. This in turn enhances the practice of a profession.

Finally, a model defines a profession. A frame of reference guides the practitioner in the immediacy of day-to-day interaction with clients. A model offers no principles that describe or prescribe the evaluation and intervention process. A model is, in a way, simply a reservoir of the collective beliefs and knowledge of a profession. A frame of reference tells the practitioner how to use or apply a portion of that knowledge to enhance the function of clients.

16/ *Summary*

Perhaps the best way to summarize this text is to return to the idea of a loop discussed in Chapter 3. The concept of loop was used to show the relationship between philosophy and practice, and where and how the occupational therapy model, frames of reference, data, and research fit into this relationship.

The occupational therapy loop is reproduced here for the reader's convenience (Fig. 1).

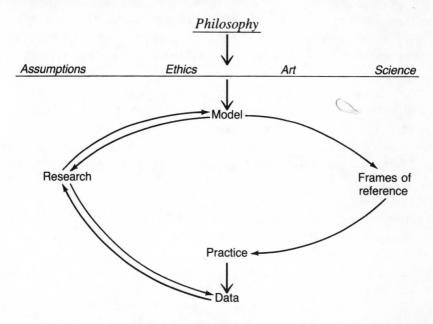

FIG. 1. The occupational therapy loop.

Similar to other professions, occupational therapy is ultimately founded on philosophy. From philosophy it derives and gains understanding of assumptions, ethics, art, and science. Over a period of time, using this philosophical foundation and the structure of professional models, occupational therapy developed the unique content of its model. This model, the content of which continues to evolve, defines the elements of occupational therapy common to the profession as a whole. The occupational therapy model is made up of statements regarding the profession's philosophical assumptions, ethical code, theoretical foundation, domain of concern, the nature of and principles for sequencing the various aspects of practice, and the profession's legitimate tools.

The various frames of reference of occupational therapy are derived from the content of the profession's model. Whereas the model defines the profession, frames of reference provide guidance for practice. Structurally, frames of reference consist of a theoretical base, function-dysfunction continuums, behavior indicative of function and dysfunction, and postulates regarding intervention. The variety of frames of reference in occupational therapy is indicative of the profession's diverse areas of specialization. It is also indicative of healthy differences in theoretical orientations relative to intervention.

Practice is based on the application of one or more frames of reference. Practice consists of evaluation and the various kinds of intervention: meeting health needs, prevention, maintenance of current function, management, and the change process. The goals of practice are influenced by the frame(s) of reference being utilized, the client's desire and potential for growth, the client's past and future expected environments, and the realistic constraints of the facility which supports the intervention process.

Practice generates both unsystematized and systematized data. Unsystematized data facilitate the formulation of tentative concepts or postulates. Systematized data derived from research are used to develop, refute, refine, or verify the theoretical systems that constitute the theoretical foundation of occupational therapy. Research findings influence initially only the theoretical foundation of occupational therapy. If a particular theory is altered through research findings, this in turn leads to alteration of those frames of reference that use that particular theoretical system. Such alteration then directly influences practice. And so there continues to be a flow through the loop which provides vitality to the practice of occupational therapy.

This text examines the form, structure, function, and component parts of occupational therapy. A configuration is proposed to serve as a point of departure and, hopefully, provide some direction for the readers' continued study of the art and science of occupational therapy.

REFERENCES

1. Ackley, N. (1962): The challenge of the sixties. *Am. J. Occup. Ther.*, 6:273–281.
2. *American Journal of Occupational Therapy* (1967): 50th Anniversary Issue, 5:259–342.
3. *American Journal of Occupational Therapy* (1977): AOTA 60th Anniversary 1917–1977 Commemorative Issue, 10:625–712.
4. *American Journal of Occupational Therapy* (1979): Specialization, 1:14–49.
5. American Occupational Therapy Association (1967): *Then—And Now: 1917–1967.* AOTA, Rockville, Md.
6. American Occupational Therapy Association (1973): *Essentials of an Accredited Program for Occupational Therapists.* AOTA, Rockville, Md.
7. American Occupational Therapy Association (1978): *Membership Handbook.* AOTA, Rockville, Md.
8. American Occupational Therapy Association (1979): The philosophical base of occupational therapy. *Am. J. Occup. Ther.*, 11:785.
9. Argyris, C., and Schon, D. A. (1974): *Theory in Practice.* Jossey-Boss Publishers, San Francisco.
10. Ayres, A. J. (1963): The development of perceptual-motor abilities: a theoretical basis for the treatment of dysfunction. *Am. J. Occup. Ther.*, 6:221–225.
11. Ayres, A. J. (1972): *Sensory Integration and Learning Disorders.* Western Psychological Services, Los Angeles.
12. Banus, B. S., editor (1979): *The Developmental Therapist.* Charles B. Slack, Thorofare, N.J.
13. Barber, B., and Wirsch, W., editors (1962): *The Sociology of Science.* The Free Press, Glencoe, Ill.
14. Benjamin, A. (1969): *The Helping Interview.* Houghton Mifflin Company, Boston.
15. Berger, M. M. (1977): *Working with People Called Patients.* Brunner Mazel, New York.
16. Bloomer, J., and Williams, S. (1979): *The Bay Area Functional Performance Evaluation. Task Oriented Assessment (TOA) and Social Interaction Scale (SIS) (Limited).* J. Bloomer and S. Williams, San Francisco.
17. Bockoven, J. S. (1971): Legacy of moral treatment—1890's to 1910. *Am. J. Occup. Ther.*, 5:223–225.
18. Borg, W. R., and Gall, M. D. (1971): *Educational Research.* David McKay Company, New York.
19. Bouchard, V. C. (1972): Hemiplegic exercise and discussion group. *Am. J. Occup. Ther.*, 7:330–331.

20. Boulding, K. G. (1968): General systems theory: skeleton of science. In: *Modern Systems Research for the Behavioral Scientist*, edited by W. Buckly, pp. 11–30. Aldine Publishing Company, Chicago.
21. Briggs, A. K., Duncombe, S. W., Howe, M. C., and Schwartzberg, S. S. (1979): *Case Simulations in Psychosocial Occupational Therapy*. F. A. Davis Company, Philadelphia.
22. Brill, A., editor (1938): *The Basic Writings of Sigmund Freud*. Random House, New York.
23. Brockema, M. C., Danz, K. H., and Schloemer, C. V. (1975): Occupational therapy in a community after care program. *Am. J. Occup. Ther.*, 1:22–27.
24. Bulger, R. J., editor (1973): *Hippocrates Revisited*. Medcom Press, New York.
25. Burke, J., and Kielhofner, G. (1977): Occupational behavior: a theory for practice. Paper presented at American Occupational Therapy Association, Pre-Conference Institute (Occupational Behavior), San Francisco.
26. Campbell, J. (1959): *The Mask of God: Primitive Mythology*. Viking Press, New York.
27. Cartwright, D., and Zander, A. (1968): *Group Dynamics: Research and Theory*. Harper & Row, New York.
28. Cassidy, H. G. (1962): *The Sciences and the Arts : A New Alliance*. Harper and Brothers, New York.
29. Clark, P. N. (1979): Human development through occupation: a philosophy and conceptual model for practice, part 2. *Am. J. Occup. Ther.*, 9:577–585.
30. Clendening, L., editor (1942): *Source Book of Medical History*. Dover Publications, New York.
31. Collins, J. (1952): *The Existentialists: A Critical Study*. Henry Regnery Company, Chicago.
32. Colman, W. (1975): Occupational therapy and child abuse. *Am. J. Occup. Ther.*, 7:412–417.
33. Combs, A. W. (1965): *The Professional Education of Teachers*. Allyn and Bacon, Boston.
34. Coser, L., and Rosenberg, B. (1957): *Sociological Theory*. The Macmillan Company, New York.
35. Cynkin, S. (1979): *Occupational Therapy: Toward Health Through Activities*. Little, Brown and Company, Boston.
36. Danto, A., and Morgenbesser, S. (1960): *Philosophy of Science*. The World Publishing Company, Cleveland.
37. Diario, K. (1971): The modern era—1960 to 1970. *Am. J. Occup. Ther.*, 5:237–242.
38. Dunning, R. E. (1973): Philosophy and occupational therapy. *Am. J. Occup. Ther.*, 1:18–23.
39. Ekstein, R., and Wallerstein, R. (1972): *The Teaching and Learning of Psychotherapy*. Basic Books, New York.
40. Ellsworth, P. (1979): Role of the occupational therapist in the promotion of health and the prevention of disability. *Am. J. Occup. Ther.*, 1:50–51.
41. Engelhardt, H. T. (1977): The meaning of therapy and the value of occupation. *Am. J. Occup. Ther.*, 10:666–672.
42. Etzioni, A., editor (1969): *The Semi-Professions and Their Organization: Teachers, Nurses, Social Workers*. Free Press, New York.

43. Fidler, G. S. (1966): Learning as a growth process : a conceptual framework for professional education. *Am. J. Occup. Ther.*, 1:1–8.
44. Fidler, G. S. (1969): The task oriented group as a context for treatment. *Am. J. Occup. Ther.*, 1:43–48.
45. Fidler, G. S. (1979): Specialization: implications for education. *Am. J. Occup. Ther.*, 1:34–45.
46. Fidler, G. S. (1979): Professional or nonprofessional. In: *Occupational Therapy: 2001 A. D.*, edited by American Occupational Therapy Association, pp. 31–36. Rockville, Md.
47. Fidler, G. S., and Fidler, J. W. (1964): *Occupational Therapy: A Communication Process in Psychiatry.* The Macmillan Company, New York.
48. Fidler, G. S., and Fidler, J. W. (1978): Doing and becoming: purposeful action and self-actualization. *Am. J. Occup. Ther.*, 5:305–310.
49. Finn, G. L. (1972): The occupational therapist in prevention programs. *Am. J. Occup. Ther.*, 2:59–66.
50. Finn, G. L. (1977): Update of Eleanor Clark Slagle lecture: the occupational therapist in prevention programs. *Am. J. Occup. Ther.*, 10:658–659.
51. Flavell, J. (1963): *The Developmental Psychology of Jean Piaget.* D. Van Nostrand Company, New York.
52. Ford, D., and Urban, H. (1963): *Systems of Psychotherapy.* John Wiley and Sons, New York.
53. Friedson, E. (1970): *Profession of Medicine.* Dodd, Mead and Company, New York.
54. Gillespie, C. C. (1960): *The Edge of Objectivity.* Princeton University Press, Princeton.
55. Gillette, N. P., and Mayer, P. R. (1968): The groups method in occupational therapy. In: *Final Report: Rehabilitation Services Administration Grant #123-T-68 for Field Consultants in Psychiatric Rehabilitation*, edited by J. Mazer, Appendix C, pp. 1–5. American Occupational Therapy Association, Rockville, Md.
56. Goldstein, P. K. (1979): Occupational therapy. In: *Preventing Physical and Mental Disabilities: Multidisciplinary Approaches*, edited by P. J. Valloluth and F. Christophos, pp. 243–258. University Park Press, Baltimore.
57. Gralewicz, A., Hill, B., and Mackinson, M. (1968): Restoration therapy: an approach to group therapy for the chronically ill. *Am. J. Occup. Ther.*, 4:294–299.
58. Greenstein, L. R. (1977): Bioethics: occupational therapy attitudes towards the prolongation of life. *Am. J. Occup. Ther.*, 2:77–80.
59. Haberman, M., and Stinnett, T. M. (1973): *Teacher Education and the New Profession of Teaching.* McCutchan Publishing Corporation, Berkeley.
60. Hare, A., Borgatta, E., and Bales, R. (1965): *Small Groups: Studies in Interaction.* Alfred A. Knopf, New York.
61. Heine, D. B. (1975): Daily living group: focus on transition from hospital to community. *Am. J. Occup. Ther.*, 10:628–630.
62. Hilgard, E., and Bower, G. (1966): *Theories of Learning.* Appleton-Century-Crofts, New York.
63. Hill, W. (1963): *Learning: A Survey of Psychological Interpretations.* Chandler Publishing Company, Scranton.
64. Holler, L. I. (1979): Remember? *Am. J. Occup. Ther.*, 8:493–499.

65. Hopkins, H. L., and Smith, H. D., editors (1978): *Willard and Spackman's Occupational Therapy.* J. B. Lippincott Company, Philadelphia.
66. Hughes, E. C., editor (1973): *Education for the Professions of Medicine, Law, Theology and Social Work.* McGraw-Hill, New York.
67. Huss, A. J. (1977): Touching with care or a caring touch. *Am. J. Occup. Ther.,* 1:11–18.
68. Jodrell, R. D., and Sanson-Fisher, R. (1975): Basic concepts of behavior modification: an experiment involving disturbed adolescent girls. *Am. J. Occup. Ther.,* 10:620–624.
69. Johnson, J. A. (1973): Occupational therapy: a model for the future. *Am. J. Occup. Ther.,* 1:1–7.
70. Johnson, J. A. (1977): Nationally speaking: representation assembly address. *Am. J. Occup. Ther.,* 9:551–554.
71. Johnson, J. A. (1977): Humanitarianism and accountability: a challenge for occupational therapy on its 60th anniversary. *Am. J. Occup. Ther.,* 10:631–637.
72. Johnson, J. A. (1978): Sixty years of progress: questions for the future. *Am. J. Occup. Ther.,* 4:209–213.
73. Jung, C. (1933): *Modern Man in Search of a Soul.* Harcourt, Brace and World, New York.
74. Jung, C. (1964): *Man and His Symbols.* Doubleday and Company, New York.
75. Kerlinger, F. N. (1973): *Foundations of Behavioral Research.* Holt, Rinehart and Winston, New York.
76. Kessler, J. F., and Froschauer, K. (1978): The soap opera: a dynamic group approach for psychiatric patients. *Am. J. Occup. Ther.,* 5:317–319.
77. Kielhofner, G. (1977): Temporal adaptation: a conceptual framework for occupational therapy. *Am. J. Occup. Ther.,* 4:235–242.
78. Kielhofner, G., and Takata, N. (1980): A study of mentally retarded persons: applied research occupational therapy. *Am. J. Occup. Ther.,* 4:252–258.
79. Kiernat, J. M. (1979): The use of life review activity with confused nursing home residents. *Am. J. Occup. Ther.,* 5:306–310.
80. King, L. J. (1974): A sensory-integrative approach to occupational therapy. *Am. J. Occup. Ther.,* 9:529–536.
81. King, L. J. (1978): Occupational therapy research in psychiatry: a perspective. *Am. J. Occup. Ther.,* 1:15–18.
82. King, L. J. (1978): Towards a science of adaptive responses. *Am. J. Occup. Ther.,* 7:429–437.
83. Kneller, G., editor (1963): *Foundations of Education.* John Wiley and Sons, New York.
84. Koch, S. (1959): *A Study of Science, Vol. II.* McGraw-Hill Company, New York.
85. Kris, E. (1952): *Psychoanalytic Explorations in Art.* International University Press, New York.
86. Kuenstler, G. (1976): A planning group for psychiatric outpatients. *Am. J. Occup. Ther.,* 10:634–639.
87. Kuhn, T. (1974): *The Structure of Scientific Revolutions.* University of Chicago Press, Chicago.

88. Laukaran, V. H. (1977): Towards a model of occupational therapy for community health. *Am. J. Occup. Ther.*, 1:71–74.

89. Lifton, W. M. (1966): *Working with Groups.* John Wiley and Sons, New York.

90. Linnell, K. E., Stechmann, A. M., and Watson, C. G. (1975): Resocialization of schizophrenic patients. *Am. J. Occup. Ther.*, 5:288–290.

91. Llorens, L. A. (1970): Facilitating growth and development: the promise of occupational therapy. *Am. J. Occup. Ther.*, 2:93–101.

92. Llorens, L. A. (1976): *Application of a Developmental Theory for Health and Rehabilitation.* American Occupational Therapy Association, Rockville, Md.

93. Lucci, J. A. (1977): *Occupational Therapy Case Studies.* Medical Examination Publishing Company, New York.

94. McGlothlin, W. (1964): *The Professional Schools.* The Center for Applied Research in Education, New York.

95. Madge, J. (1962): *The Origins of Scientific Sociology.* The Free Press, New York.

96. Manam, G. D. (1973): *The Group Approach in Nursing Practice.* C. V. Mosby Company, St. Louis.

97. Mann, W., Godfrey, M. E., and Dowd, E. T. (1973): The use of group counseling procedures in the rehabilitation of spinal cord injured patients. *Am. J. Occup. Ther.*, 2:73–77.

98. Mann, W., and Sobsey (1975): Feeding programs for the institutionalized mentally retarded. *Am. J. Occup. Ther.*, 471–474.

99. Marx, M., and Hillix, W. (1963): *Systems and Theories in Psychology.* McGraw-Hill Company, New York.

100. Maslow, A. H. (1966): *The Psychology of Science.* Henry Regnery Company, Chicago.

101. Mazer, J. L., Fidler, G. S., Kovalenko, L. J., and Overly, K. (1970): *Exploring How a Think Feels.* American Occupational Therapy Association, Rockville, Md.

102. Menks, F., Sittler, S., Weaver, D., and Yanou, B. (1977): A psychogeriatric activity group in a rural community. *Am. J. Occup. Ther.*, 6:376–384.

103. Meyer, A. (1977): The philosophy of occupational therapy. *Am. J. Occup. Ther.*, 10:639–642.

104. Mills, T. M. (1967): *The Sociology of Small Groups.* Prentice-Hall, Englewood Cliffs, N.J.

105. Moore, J. C. (1977): Individual differences and the art of therapy. *Am. J. Occup. Ther.*, 10:663–665.

106. Moore, O. K., and Anderson, A. R. (1968): Some principles for the design of clarifying educational environments. Learning Research and Development Center, University of Pittsburgh, Pre-print no. 32. Pittsburgh.

107. Moore, W. E. (1970): *The Professions: Roles and Rules.* Russell Sage Foundation, New York.

108. Mosey, A. C. (1970): *Three Frames of Reference for Mental Health.* Charles B. Slack, Thorofare, N.J.

109. Mosey, A. C. (1971): Involvement in the rehabilitation movement 1942 to 1960. *Am. J. Occup. Ther.*, 5:234–236.

110. Mosey, A. C. (1973): Meeting health needs. *Am. J. Occup. Ther.*, 1:14–17.

111. Mosey, A. C. (1973): *Activities Therapy.* Raven Press, New York.

112. Mosey, A. C. (1974): An alternative: the biopsychosocial model. *Am. J. Occup. Ther.*, 3:137–140.
113. Murphy, E. A. (1976): *The Logic of Medicine.* The Johns Hopkins University Press, Baltimore.
114. Nagel, E. (1961): *The Structure of Science.* Harcourt, Brace and World, New York.
115. Nidditch, P. H., editor (1968): *The Philosophy of Science.* Oxford University Press, London.
116. *Occupational Therapy Newspaper* (1979): Highlights of actions taken by the representative assembly, 6:1.
117. Ostrow, P. C. (1980): The care and feeding of theories. *Am. J. Occup. Ther.*, 4:272–273.
118. Parson, T. (1951): *The Social System.* The Free Press, New York.
119. Parsons, T., and Bales, R. F. (1955): *Family, Socialization and Interaction Process.* The Free Press, New York.
120. Piaget, J. (1952): *The Origin of Intelligence in Children.* International Universities Press, New York.
121. Popper, K. P. (1972): *Objective Knowledge: An Evolutionary Approach.* Oxford University Press, London.
122. Posthuma, B. W., and Posthuma, A. B. (1972): The effect of small-group experience on occupational therapy students. *Am. J. Occup. Ther.*, 8:415–418.
123. Pratt, C. (1948): *The Logic of Modern Psychology.* The Macmillan Company, New York.
124. Professional Examination Service (1975): *Development of Occupational Therapy Proficiency.* New York.
125. Rance, C., and Price, A. (1973): Poetry as a group project. *Am. J. Occup. Ther.*, 5:252–255.
126. Randall, J. H., and Buchler, J. (1970): *Philosophy: An Introduction.* Barnes and Noble, New York.
127. Reed, K., and Sanderson, S. R. (1980): *Concepts of Occupational Therapy.* Williams & Wilkins, Baltimore.
128. Reilly, M. (1962): Occupational therapy can be one of the greatest ideas of 20th century medicine. *Am. J. Occup. Ther.*, 1:1–9.
129. Reilly, M. (1969): The educational process. *Am. J. Occup. Ther.*, 4:299–307.
130. Reilly, M. (1971): The modernization of occupational therapy. *Am. J. Occup. Ther.*, 5:243–246.
131. Reilly, M., editor (1974): *Play as Exploratory Learning.* Sage Publications, Beverly Hills.
132. Report of the task force on social issues (1972): *Am. J. Occup. Ther.*, 7:332–359.
133. Rerek, M. D. (1971): The depression years—1929 to 1941. *Am. J. Occup. Ther.*, 5:231–233.
134. Rogers, C. R. (1961): *On Becoming a Person.* Houghton Mifflin Company, Boston.
135. Rood, M. S. (1958): Everyone counts. *Am. J. Occup. Ther.*, 6:326–329.
136. Rosenberg, C. E., editor (1979): *Healing and History.* Dawson, Science History Publications, New York.
137. Rubenstein, R., and Lasswell, H. (1966): *The Sharing of Power in a Psychiatric Hospital.* Yale University Press, New Haven.

138. Runes, D. D., editor (1962): *Living Schools of Philosophy*. Littlefield, Adams and Company, Paterson, N.J.

139. Sahakian, W. S. (1968): *Outline: History of Philosophy*. Barnes and Noble, New York.

140. Samson, E. E., and Marthas, M. S. (1977): *Group Process for the Health Professions*. John Wiley and Sons, New York.

141. Schein, E. H. (1972): *Professional Education*. McGraw-Hill, New York.

142. Schulman, E. D. (1974): *Intervention in Human Services*. C. V. Mosby Company, St. Louis.

143. Searles, H. T. (1960): *The Non-human Environment*. International Universities Press, New York.

144. Selltiz, C., Wrightsman, L. S., and Cook, S. W. (1976): *Research Methods in Social Relations*. Holt, Rinehart, and Winston, New York.

145. Shannon, P. D. (1977): The derailment of occupational therapy. *Am. J. Occup. Ther.*, 4:229–234.

146. Shannon, P. D. (1978): American Occupational Therapy Association project to identify the philosophy of occupational therapy. Memorandum addressed to curriculum directors.

147. Shryock, R. H. (1947): *The Development of Modern Medicine*. Alfred A. Knopf, New York.

148. Sieg, K. W. (1974): Applying the behavioral model to the occupational therapy model. *Am. J. Occup. Ther.*, 7:421–428.

149. Simon, J. L. (1978): *Basic Research in Social Sciences*. Random House, New York.

150. Stabbing, L. S. (1952): *A Modern Elementary Logic*. University Paperbacks, Methuen, England.

151. Stattel, F. M. (1956): Equipment designed for occupational therapy. *Am. J. Occup. Ther.*, 1:194–198.

152. Stein, J., and Urdang, L., editors (1966): *The Random House Dictionary of the English Language*. Random House, New York.

153. Sullivan, H. S. (1953): *The Interpersonal Theory of Psychiatry*. W. W. Norton and Company, New York.

154. Trombly, C. A., and Scott, A. D. (1977): *Occupational Therapy for Physical Dysfunction*. Williams & Wilkins, Baltimore.

155. Ullmann, L. P., and Krasner, L., editors (1965): *Case Studies in Behavior Modification*. Holt, Rinehart, and Winston, New York.

156. Von Bartolanfly, L. (1968): General systems theory: a critical review. In: *Modern Systems Research for the Behavioral Scientist*, edited by W. Buckly, pp. 11–30. Aldine Publishing Company, Chicago.

157. Walizer, M. H., and Wienir, P. L. (1978): *Research Methods and Analysis: Searching for Relationships*. Harper & Row, Publishers, New York.

158. Weber, J. W. (1978): Chaining strategies for teaching sequential motor tasks to mentally retarded adults. *Am. J. Occup. Ther.*, 6:385–389.

159. Wells, C. A. (1976): Ethics in conflict: yesterday's standards—outdated guide for tomorrow. *Am. J. Occup. Ther.*, 1:44–47.

160. West, W. L. (1968): Professional responsibilities in times of change. *Am. J. Occup. Ther.*, 1:9–15.

161. West, W. L. (1979): Professional unity. *Am. J. Occup. Ther.*, 1:40–49.

162. West, W. (1979): Historical perspectives. In: *Occupational Therapy: 2001 A. D.*, edited by American Occupational Therapy Association, pp. 9–17. Rockville, Md.

163. Whitaker, S. D., and Lieberman, A. (1964): *Psychotherapy Through the Group Process*. Atherton Press, New York.

164. Williams, R., and Bener, N. (1976): The day hospital at the Burke Rehabilitation Center. *Am. J. Occup. Ther.*, 5:293.

165. Wollmer, H., and Mills, D., editors (1966): *Professionalism*. Prentice-Hall, Englewood Cliffs, N.J.

166. Woodride, H. H. (1971): The development of occupational therapy—1910 to 1929. *Am. J. Occup. Ther.*, 5:226–230.

167. Yalom, I. D. (1975): *The Theory and Practice of Group Psychotherapy*. Basic Books, New York.

168. Yerxa, E. J. (1967): Authentic occupational therapy. *Am. J. Occup. Ther.*, 1:1–9.

169. Yerxa, E. J. (1979): The philosophical base of occupational therapy. In: *Occupational Therapy: 2001 A.D.*, edited by American Occupational Therapy Association, pp. 26–30. Rockville, Md.

170. Zilboorg, G. (1941): *A History of Medical Psychology*. W. W. Norton and Company, New York.

171. Zwieg, P. (1980): Review of *The White Lantern*, by E. S. Connell. *The New York Times Book Review*, July 20.

Subject Index

Abstract definition, 35–36
Academic discipline versus profession, 124
Acquisitional frames of reference, *see* Frames of reference, acquisitional
Actions, voluntary, ethics and, 20
Activity(ies)
  purposeful, *see* Purposeful activity(ies)
  specific knowledge of, 118
Activity analysis and synthesis, 113–118
  definition of, 114
  generic, 115
  restricted, 116–118
Activity group(s), 107–113
  constructive use of nonhuman environment in, 109
  as laboratory, 108
  structure and organization and, 108–109
  types of, 110–113
Addiction, 11
Administrator, occupational therapist as, 13
Adolescents, 10
Aesthetics, 21–25; *see also* Art
Age-appropriate skills, 148
American Occupational Therapy Association, 66
American Occupational Therapy Delegate Assembly, 58
Analytical frames of reference, *see* Frames of reference, analytical
Anxiety, 11
  conflict and, 145–146
  nonhuman environment as source of, 92–93
Art, 21–25, 158
  definition of, 23
  in theoretical foundation of occupational therapy, 73

Art of practice, 4, 21–25
  conscious use of self and, 96
  definition of, 22
Arthritis, 12
Arts and crafts, 102
Assumptions
  of analytical frames of reference, 145
  of developmental frames of reference, 147
  of philosophy, 17–19, 158
  of science, 28
Attitude of client, 7

Base of frame of reference, 133
Behaviours indicative of function and dysfunction, *see* Function/dysfunction continuums
Biofeedback, 55
Biological deficit, 7
Biological sciences in theoretical foundation of occupational therapy, 72
Biological stress, 7
Biological trauma, 7
Biopsychosocial model as integrative idea for occupational therapy, 121
Burns, 12

Cancer, 12
Cardiovascular disease, 11
Care of chronically impaired individual, 59
Cause of illness, 80
Centrality of activities, 112–113
Cerebral palsy, children with, 10
Cerebral vascular accident, 11
Change process, 85
  frames of reference and, 144
Child abuse, 11
  ethical issues of, 20

Children, occupational therapists' work
with, 9–10
Choice, personal, 61
Chores, 102–103
Circumscribed focus of activity group,
113
Classroom tests, 117
Client
definition of, 6
knowledge, skills, and attitudes of, 7
occupational therapist and, 4–5
rights of, 5
Client population, 9–12
Code of ethics, see Ethical code
Cognitive function, 75
Collaborative process, occupational
therapy as, 5
Collagen diseases, 85–86
Common themes in occupational
therapy, 120–123
Concepts
exclusivity of, 34–35
of theory, 32–33, 35
types of, 34
Conceptual framework of activity
analysis and synthesis, 113
Conceptualization, 33
Concurrent activity group, 112
Conflict, repression of, 145–147
Conscious use of self, 95–97
versus spontaneous response to
another person, 96
Constructs, 34
Consultant, occupational therapist as, 13
Continuum, definition of, 116; see also
Function-dysfunction continuums
Core of domain of concern, 74–75
Correlative postulate, 37
Course of illness, 81
Critical evaluation of facts of experience,
16
Cultural environment, 78
Cultural symbols, 104, 105

Data
in occupational therapy loop, 43
ordering of, 30–40
research and, 44

statistical analysis of, 39
systematized and unsystematized, 158
Defense mechanisms, 60
Deficit, biological, 7
Definition(s)
by example, 36
of model, 49–57
structural component of theory as, 35
types of, 35–36
Depression, 11
Descriptive definition, 36
Developmental frames of reference, see
Frames of reference,
developmental
Disease, 80
Domain of concern
frame of reference and, 130
of occupational therapy, 74–79
of profession, 51–52, 74
Dynamic theory, 134
Dysfunction, behavior indicative of, 82,
138–140

Education of occupational therapists,
14–15
Educator, occupational therapist as, 15
Elderly individuals, 11–12
Emotionally disturbed children, 10
Empathy and sympathy, difference
between, 24
Environment
external, postulates regarding intervention and, 142
human and nonhuman, individual's
interaction with, 61–62
nonhuman, 8, 9, 78–79, 89–95
constructive use of, 109
definition of, 89
as foundation of human nature, 93
individual's interaction with, 61–62
natural tension and, 94
performance components and, 91–
92
quality of life and, 92
scientist's concern for, 25
security and, 90
self-understanding and, 91
as source of anxiety, 92–93

as source of pleasure, 92
as occupational therapy's domain of concern, 78–79
self and, differentiation between, 90
Ethical code, 17
functions of, 21
of occupational therapy, 64–70
Ethics, 19–21, 158
social sciences and, 20
Evaluation, 158
definition of, 86–87
restricted conceptual framework and, 116–117
Evaluation procedures, frames of reference and, 139–140
Evaluation type of activity group, 110
Evaluative criteria for theory, 38–39
Everyday life, purposeful activities in, 103

Field theory, 49
Field work, 14
First premises of philosophical assumptions, 18
Frames of reference, 154–156, 158
acquisitional, 150–152
function-dysfunction continuums of, 151
analytical, 144–146
theoretical base of, 145
base of, 133
behavior indicative of function or dysfunction and, 138–140
change process and, 144
definition of, 41–42, 129–132
developmental, 147–150
postulates regarding change in, 149
theoretical base of, 148
domain of concern and, 130
dynamic and static theories in, 134–135
function-dysfunction continuums and, 130, 136–138
functions of, 130
for professional model, 41
relationship of model to, 155–156
relationship of theory to, 154–155
selection of, 131

standardized evaluation procedures and 139–140
structure of, 133–143
theoretical base of, 127, 133–136
types of, 144–151
differences between, 152–153
as word picture, 130
Function and dysfunction, behaviors indicative of, 82, 138–140
Function-dysfunction continuums, 136–138, 158
acquisitional frame of reference and, 151
developmental frame of reference and, 149
frame of reference and, 130, 136–138
Functional definition, 36

Games
of chance, 102
as purposeful activities, 101
of strategy, 102
Generic activity analysis and synthesis, 115
Group, see Activity group(s)
Group interaction skill, function-dysfunction continuum and, 136
Growth and development
as integrative idea for occupational therapy, 122
purposeful activities and, 99

Health model as alternative to medical model, 121
Health needs, 82–84, 158
definition of, 83
Hierarchical postulates, 37
Hippocratic Oath, 64–65, 69
Hypotheses, use of, 26–7

Idiosyncratic symbols, 105
Immediacy of events in activity group, 113
Information gathering within profession, 54–55
Insight, development of, 147, 152
Instrumental type of activity group, 112

Integrative ideas for occupational
   therapy, 119–125
Intervention, 86
   postulates regarding, 141–143
Intervention process, 82–86
Intimacy between occupational therapist
   and client, 4
Irrational behavior, unconscious conflict
   and, 146

Kant, 17–18
Kepler, 31
Kidney dialysis, 12
Knowledge
   of client, 7
   creation of versus application of, 124
   scientific, communication, of, 29

Labeling, 33–34
Laboratory, activity group as, 108
Learning
   through activity group, 108
   definition of, 98
   as essence of purposeful activity, 100
   through imitation, 44
Learning disabled children and adults,
   55, 56
Legitimate tools
   of occupational therapy, 89–118
   of profession, 52
Life tasks, 6–7
Loop
   occupational therapy, 42, 43, 157
   between philosophy and practice, 41–
   45

Maintenance of function, 59, 85, 157
Management in occupational therapy
   practice, 86, 158
Mead, Margaret, 101
Meaningful existence, right to, 59
Medical model, 50, 80
   versus occupational therapy model, 50,
   121
Medical practice, sequence of, 81
Medicine
   domain of concern in, 74
   occupational therapy and, 73

different philosophical assumptions
   of, 19
   theoretical foundation of, 71
Meeting health needs, *see* Health needs
Method of science, 28–30
Meyers, Adolph, 121
Model, *see also* Professional model
   as basis for practice, 41
   definition of, 41, 49–50
   frames of reference and, 153–154
   medical, *see* Medical model
   for occupational therapy, 42
   sociologists' definition of, 49–50
   structure of, 51–52
Moore and Anderson, 101–102
Moral behavior, 64
Muscle strength, function-dysfunction
   continuum and, 136

Natural purposeful activities, 106–107
Neurological diseases, 85–86
Neuromuscular function, 75
Nonhuman environment, *see* Environ-
   ment, nonhuman
Norms, determination of, 140

Observable events, 31
Occupational versus profession, 19–20
Occupational performance, 7
   as integrative idea for occupational
   therapy, 122
Occupational therapist
   client and, 4–5
   education of, 14–15
   roles of, 13–15
Occupational therapy
   definition of, 3, 15
   ethical code of, 64–70
   philosophical assumptions of, 58–62
   profession of, 3–9
   specialization in, 119
   theoretical foundation of, 71–73
Occupational therapy loop, 42, 43, 157
Occupational therapy model versus
   medical model, 50
Operational definition, 36
Ordering of data, 30–40

Paradigm
  concept of, 123–125
  definition of, 123
Pathology, 80
Patient, definition of, 6
Performance components
  of analytical frames of reference, 145
  of domain of concern of occupational therapy, 74
  nonhuman environment and, 91–92
Personal choice, 61
Personal potential, 61
Philosophers
  concerns of, 16
  of science, concerns of, 27–28
Philosophical assumptions, 17–19
  as integrative idea for occupational therapy, 121
  of occupational therapy, 59–63
  of profession, 18–19
  versus scientific theories, 18
Philosophical Base of Occupational Therapy, statement of, 59–63
Philosophical origin of occupational therapy, 16–40
Philosophy
  definition of, 16
  practice and, 157
    loop relationship between, 41–45
  schools of, 18
  science and, 17, 26–27, 158
Pierce, Charles S., 18
Play
  inherent need for, 62
  as purposeful activity, 101
Pleasure, nonhuman environment as source of, 92
Pledge and Creed for Occupational Therapists, 65–66
Postulates, 36–37
  regarding change, 149
  regarding intervention, 141–143, 151, 158
  types of, 36–37
Potential, personal, 61
Practice, 158
  art of, see Art of practice

of occupational therapy, aspects of, 80–88
  sequence of, 87–88
  philosophy and, 157
  loop relationship between, 41–45
Prediction, purpose of theory and, 31
Prevention
  of illness, 80–81
  in occupational therapy practice, 84, 158
Primary group, 107
Principles of Occupational Therapy Ethics, 66–69
Profession
  versus academic discipline, 124
  code of ethics of, 22
  domain of concern of, 51–52, 74
  information gathering within, 54–55
  legitimate tools of, 52
  versus occupation, 19–20
  occupational therapy as, 3–9
  philosophical assumptions of, 18–19
  sense of identity of, 53
  theoretical foundation of, 51, 71
Professional model, 158; see also Model
  changes in, 55
  evolution of, 44, 52–57
    restraints on, 55–57
  frame of reference and, 130
  origin of, 44
  periodic reassessment of, 54
  statement of content of, 53
  structure of, 51–52
Prognosis of illness, 81
Psychodynamics, 146
Psychological function, 75–76
Psychological stress, 8
Psychology in theoretical foundation of occupational therapy, 72
Pulmonary deficit, 11
Purposeful activity(ies), 99–107
  definition of, 62
  in everyday life, 103
  games as, 101
  as integrative idea for occupational therapy, 122
  learning as essence of, 100
  natural, 106–107

observation of, 103
play as, 101
versus random activities, 99
realistic nature of, 104
simulated, 106, 107
symbolic nature of, 104
Puzzle solving, 101–102

Quality of life, nonhuman environment
    and, 92
Quantitative postulate, 37

Radial nerve, severance of, 10–11
Random activity, 62
    versus purposeful activity, 99
Rapport, 9
    conscious use of self and, 96
Realistic nature of purposeful activities,
    104
Recreation/leisure, 77
Reilly, Mary, 101, 102, 123
Research, data and, 44
research projects, occupational therapists
    in, 14
Resident, definition of, 6
Rest, inherent need for, 62
Restricted activity analysis and
    synthesis, 116–118
Retarded children, 10
Roles of occupational therapist, 13–15
Rules of science, 28

Schools of philosophy, 18
Science, 25–28
    method of, 28–30
    modern and early, differences between,
        26–27
    occupational therapy as, 4, 5
    philosophers of, 27–28
    philosophy and, 17, 26–27, 158
Scientific findings, provisional nature of,
    29–30
Scientific inquiry, 28–29
    ordering of data and, 30
Scientific knowledge, communication of,
    29
Scientific theories versus philosophical

assumptions, 18
Searles, Harold, 90
Security, nonhuman environment and, 90
Selected theories in occupational
    therapy, 4
Self
    conscious use of, 95–97
    environment and, differentiation
        between, 90
Self-doubt in occupational therapy, 119–
    120
Self-understanding, nonhuman
    environment and, 91
Sense of identity, professional, 53
Sensory integration, 75
Sequelae of illness, 81
Sequence
    of aspects of practice, 87–88
    of medical practice, 81
Sequencing, principles of, 80
Settings for work, 12–13
Sheltered workshop program, 12
Sign
    definition of, 104
    of illness, 80
Simple concepts, 34
Simulated purposeful activities, 106–107
Skills of client, 7
Skinner's theory of operant conditioning,
    55, 98
Slagle, Eleanor Clark, 121
Social environment, 78
Social nature of species, 60
Social sciences, ethics and, 20
Socialization process, purposeful
    activities and, 101
Sociological stress, 8
Sociologists' definition of model, 49–50
Sociology in theoretical foundation of
    occupational therapy, 72–73
Spatial postulate, 37
Specialization in occupational therapy,
    119
Splinter skills, 148
Spontaneous responses to another
    person, 96
Stage-specific maturation of species, 60
Static theory, 134

Statistical analysis of data, 39
Stress, 7–8
Structural components of theory, 32–38
Structure
    activity group and, 108–109
    of frame of reference, 133–143
    of professional model, 51–52
Symbol(s)
    cultural, 104, 105
    definition of, 104
    idiosyncratic, 105
    unconscious conflict and, 146
    universal, 104, 105
Symbolic nature of purposeful activities,
    104
Sympathy and empathy, difference
        between, 24
Symptom of illness, 80

Task Force on Ethics, 66
Task-oriented activity group, 110–111
Teaching, definition of, 98
Teaching-learning process, 97–99
Temporal adaptation, 77–78
Temporal postulate, 37
Tension, nonhuman environment and, 94
Theoretical foundation
    of frame of reference, 133–136
        analytical, 145
        developmental, 148
    of occupational therapy, 71–73, 158
        as integrative idea, 121
    of profession, 51, 71
Theory, 30–40
    concepts of, 32–33, 35

descriptive nature of, 154
evaluative criteria for, 38–39
frames of reference and, 154–155
functions of, misconceptions about,
    31–32
purpose of, 30–31
refinement of, 30
refutation of, 30
structural components of, 32–38
Tools, legitimate, *see* Legitimate tools
Traditions of science, 28
Transference in analytic frames of
        reference, 146, 152
Trauma, biological, 7
Treatment of illness, 81

Unconscious conflict, 145–146
Unconscious content, symbols and, 145–
    146
Universal symbols, 104, 105

Variables, 34
Visual form and space perception,
        function-dysfunction continuum
        and, 136
Voluntary actions, ethics and, 20

War injury, 12
Word picture, frame of reference as, 130
Work, 77
    inherent need for, 62
    settings for, 12–13

Zweig, Paul, 40